WIN THE BATTLE
AGAINST
BACK PAIN:
AN INTEGRATED MIND-BODY APPROACH

D0097128

MICHAEL S. SINEL, M.D.
WILLIAM W. DEARDORFF, Ph.D.
THEODORE B. GOLDSTEIN, M.D.

A DELL TRADE PAPERBACK

A DELL TRADE PAPERBACK

Published by
Dell Publishing
a division of
Bantam Doubleday Dell Publishing Group, Inc.
1540 Broadway
New York, New York 10036

Library of Congress Cataloging in Publication Data

Sinel, Michael S.
Win the battle against back pain : an integrated mind-body approach / Michael S. Sinel, William W. Deardorff, Theodore B. Goldstein.
p.   cm.
Includes bibliographical references and index.
ISBN 0-440-50705-7
1. Backache—Popular works.   I. Deardorff, William W.
II. Goldstein, Theodore B.   III. Title.
RD771.B217S57   1996
617.5′64—dc20   96-4307
                                                          CIP

Printed in the United States of America

Published simultaneously in Canada

October 1996

10 9 8 7 6 5 4 3 2 1

CRITICAL RAVES FOR
WIN THE BATTLE AGAINST BACK PAIN

"As a longtime back-pain sufferer, I was told never to pick up anything heavy. Well, this book isn't heavy, but it's the best thing you'll ever pick up if you just read it. Thanks to these prominent doctors, I sat painlessly and read it thoroughly. So should you!"
—*Neil Simon*, playwright

"In my family, we live with the issue of back pain every day. We are winning the battle because of an approach to its containment and treatment as presented in this book. THIS IS A MUST READ FOR PEOPLE WITH BACK PAIN."
—*Gerry Spence, Esq.*, attorney and bestselling author

"With the knowledge that comes only from experience and the wisdom that comes from reflection, this book provides a balanced view of back pain, assessing its causes and treatments. The object is to make you, the patient, an understanding contributor to your own recovery. A human and thoughtful response to one of the most common sources of human suffering. If you are contemplating any kind of back-pain treatment, THIS BOOK IS AN ESSENTIAL GUIDE TO YOUR REHABILITATION—A MUST READ."
—*David Viscott, M.D.*, bestselling author

"A wealth of well-documented information and practical advice on back pain, put together by an experienced team of clinicians working closely together. IT WILL BE OF IMMENSE VALUE TO PATIENTS AND HEALTH PROFESSIONALS ALIKE."
—*Kn Kit Hui, M.D., F.A.C.P.*, director, UCLA Center for East-West Medicine

Dear Reader:

The information, advice, and suggestions contained in this book are based on the latest scientific evidence as well as on our extensive clinical experience working in a multidisciplinary spine institute. Even so, this book is not intended as a substitute for the services of a physician. If you decide to follow any advice or suggestions presented in this book, you must assume full responsibility and do so at your sole discretion.

Since we cannot be aware of your unique back-pain problem, it is important for you to work with your doctor, who is familiar with your individual case. If the information in this book differs from what you have been told about your particular condition, those differences should be discussed with your doctor until you are satisfied that you are obtaining good care.

Sincerely,

Michael S. Sinel, M.D.
William W. Deardorff, Ph.D.
Theodore B. Goldstein, M.D.

CONTENTS

CONTENTS

PART IV
THE POWER OF THE MIND IN BACK PAIN

PREFACE

Over the past few years we have observed a tremendous number of back-pain patients who have been misdiagnosed and mistreated by a variety of health professionals, often leading to unnecessary disability. A large number of patients who come to our spine clinic have already seen several physicians and other health care professionals for their complaint of back pain. This has afforded us the opportunity to make the observation that the great majority of back-pain sufferers are over-rested, overmedicated, and overoperated, often due to a lack of knowledge by the professionals advising them.

The lack of agreement on the diagnosis and treatment of such a common ailment is unparalleled. This has created an environment in which practitioners of all sorts, from physicians in many specialties, to chiropractors, to a variety of other allied health professionals, have entered the arena in the battle against back pain. All of these professionals bring with them a different approach.

As is to be expected, significant controversy exists between the various practitioners as to the best treatment for back pain. This causes patients afflicted with back pain to have a very difficult and confusing choice, which can mean the difference between good care and poor care, and useless treatment, which can be harmful.

This book is written in an attempt to help back-pain sufferers approach their problem in the most healthy, useful, and safe manner possible. It will inform you as to the agreed-upon, although still incomplete, knowledge about back pain that exists today. This knowledge can be crucial in helping you avoid the often useless, unnecessary, and potentially harmful treatment all too commonly recommended. The authors have had the unique opportunity to have been trained by, and practiced with, many of the world-renowned leaders in several medical specialties and allied health fields dedicated to treating back pain. Our present clinical practice allows us personally to evaluate and treat the complete spectrum of back-pain problems from day one of an acute disc herniation, at one extreme, to chronic back pain of twenty-five years' duration with multiple failed surgeries at another.

We see over 150 new patients per month at our spine clinic, which is composed of orthopedists, neurosurgeons, physiatrists, psychologists, physical and occupational therapists, and exercise physiologists. We also interact closely with neurologists, chiropractors, anesthesiologists, and others in the surrounding community, who provide care for patients with back pain. We all agree that the amount of misinformation about back pain is astounding.

In such a rapidly changing field it is critical that we continue to seek out new knowledge about back pain, and we strongly encourage the reader to do the same. For that reason we have provided a bibliography of readings for most topics presented in the book. It is beyond the scope of this book to provide exhaustive information on back pain, as there are libraries full of such information. Rather it is our intent to provide you with the most up-to-date and useful information, as well as a means of evaluating this information as it pertains to you. We hope this book helps you avoid the frequent and often unnecessary suffering that often accompanies back pain.

Michael S. Sinel, M.D.
William W. Deardorff, Ph.D.
Theodore B. Goldstein, M.D.

PART I

YOU AND YOUR BACK

CHAPTER 1

WHY A BOOK ABOUT BACK PAIN?

This book was developed out of our frustration and desperation in treating back-pain sufferers. The frustration came from seeing how our cultural attitudes have influenced back pain and how medical practice has managed (or rather mismanaged) this problem. In the end we all suffer as a result of this mismanagement. Society suffers from exorbitant costs associated with back pain. Families suffer from the stress of living with the person in pain, who may be unable to work and socialize and may even have a significant change in personality. But most importantly, you, the person with back pain, suffers, not only from the pain but also from fear of doing activities you enjoy, financial stress, relationship problems, and a bewildering array of high-tech medical approaches of often unproven efficacy. *This book was written for you.*

In our practice we see back pain of all types and duration. We see back pain that starts with a car accident, work injury, or other trauma. We see men and women of all ages, racial groups, and occupations who suffer from back pain. The pain may have been with them for as short a time as one day or as long as thirty years. In an alarming number of cases we hear tales of inappropriate treatment, incorrect information, and unnecessary surgeries.

Dr. Wilbert Fordyce, professor emeritus at the University of Washington and cofounder of the world's first pain center, has termed this process the medicalization of suffering. As we shall see in this book, suffering occurs when a situation threatens the wellness and intactness of a person. Suffering happens when a person anticipates a severe threat of loss in the present or future. *Suffering is the emotional reaction to a threat.* Back pain is perceived as a threat to our well-being and can elicit severe suffering, which in turn makes the pain worse. Ironically suffering is often due to misinformation. For instance you may have thoughts such as the following:

> "My doctor told me to let pain be my guide, but the pain guides me to do nothing."
> "The pain really scares me."
> "I must find the reason for this pain."
> "If I move the wrong way, my pain will get worse."
> "I can't live with this pain."
> "I'll never be able to lead a normal life."
> "There must be something seriously wrong with my spine, otherwise the pain would be gone."
> "Nobody understands my pain."

These thoughts, however subtle, can have a profound effect on your pain. In addition they can cause you to suffer from increased emotional distress.

The medical and legal professions often increase a person's suffering with back pain. In the vast majority of cases suffering is unnecessary, preventable, and reversible. We have seen this proven time and time again in our clinical practice. In addition, research and international statistics in this area have documented this over the past ten years. However, the medical profession as a whole only receives this information in limited amounts and often does not put it into practice. It is for this reason that we have decided to get the information directly to the people, like you, with back pain.

The Scientific Evidence
This book is based on the latest scientific findings about back pain. It is also based on our extensive clinical experience putting these principles into practice. Much of this information comes from several landmark studies and research reviews. These are the Quebec Task Force on Spinal Disorders, the Boeing Study, the National Health and Nutrition Examination

Survey (NHANES II), and the recently released clinical practice guidelines on back pain compiled by the Agency for Health Care Policy and Research (AHCPR) of the U.S. government. Many other studies are also discussed, as well as findings from our clinical experience treating hundreds of back-pain patients.

The Quebec Task Force on Spinal Disorders was commissioned in 1983 to study spine problems in the workplace. Members of the task force included experts in spinal disorders from all over the world. The study took over two years to complete and included a review of over seven thousand research articles from the ten years prior to the study. In addition the task force looked at back problems in three thousand injured workers from the Quebec area. The primary concern was how spine problems were being diagnosed and treated, and whether the treatment was having any benefit. It was also commissioned to make recommendations to improve the quality of treatment for back problems. Even though this study concluded several years ago, most of the recommendations are not put into practice by the medical profession in general.

The Boeing Study is probably one of the most important investigations of back pain. It involved studying 3,020 employees of the Boeing Aircraft Company in Seattle over many years. The employees were given many physical and psychological tests and then monitored to see who would develop back-pain problems. Of the original group 279 employees reported disabling back problems over the subsequent four years. The study was able to show that psychological stress (such as job dissatisfaction) predicted back-pain problems more than any of the physical measures (physical examination, height, weight, flexibility, and strength, etc.). This was important in showing that back pain is a complex phenomenon.

The NHANES II study looked at 27,801 subjects across the United States. Of these, 10,404 reported they had had an incident of low back pain in their lifetime. In addition 1,516 reported on their use of health care professionals for their back-pain problem, and information was gathered about the types of treatments administered, the percentage of those who thought that the treatment helped, and the percentage of those still using the treatment. The results of this survey are presented throughout this book.

The AHCPR was established in 1989 to enhance the quality and effectiveness of health care services. As such the agency develops practice guidelines in a number of medical areas. The guidelines for evaluation and treatment of back pain were released in 1994. These are the results of a research panel reviewing over ten thousand scientific studies on the evaluation and treatment of back pain. The panel looked at which studies were conducted appropriately using a critical-review approach and then summarized which treatments were shown to be effective in back pain and which were not. This resulted in evaluation and treatment guidelines, many of which will become the standard for the medical profession over the next several years. This book will give you that up-to-date information in an easy-to-understand format so that you can determine whether your treatment is being conducted along the lines of accepted scientific knowledge or not.

A Typical Case Example: Lingering Back Pain

In industrialized countries treatment for back pain proceeds along a fairly predictable course. Surprisingly, new research shows that the treatment you receive for your back pain may be more disabling and dangerous than the back pain itself.

Back pain is an individual experience and it impacts everyone differently. Whether you have experienced a single back-pain episode or a recurrent back-pain problem, you can probably relate to the following typical scenario. It is a fictitious case example based on a combination of many cases. You may find your situation falls near the beginning of the case scenario or near the end. Either way it is important to understand these events so that you can stop being victimized by the medical system and begin to take control of your life.

Whether your pain started with a specific event (for example an auto or work injury) or just seemed slowly to become worse and worse, you probably tried to ignore the pain, hoping it would go away. You may try bed rest, aspirin, and a hot-water bottle. You may also try to "take it easy" to protect your back and relieve the pain. When that fails to work, or only works for a short time, you go to your family doctor or internist. Your family doctor most likely continues with "conservative" treatment. You may be prescribed medicines (pain, anti-inflammatories, or muscle relaxants) along with a mild home-exercise program. You are told to "let pain be your guide" and are sent on your way. Still the pain lingers.

As time goes on, you become more concerned about the pain. It has never lasted this long before. You begin to baby your back for fear the pain means you are damaging something in your spine. Finally you return to your family doctor, who sends you to a specialist. Statistics show that in most cases this will be an orthopedist. You may have an examination and are prescribed physical therapy along with more medicine. The physical therapy consists of hot packs, cold packs, ultrasound, massage, and light exercise. It feels good while you are at the clinic, but the pain returns soon after each treatment session. It is hard to say whether the treatment is actually helping or not. You wonder what is wrong with your back that would cause such prolonged pain. You reason that if your back hurts, it must need rest and protection. You get prescribed a brace to wear, which feels good for a while but when you take it off, the pain is worse.

You return to the orthopedist, who feels it is time for some diagnostic tests. You have an MRI of your spine. The results come in and your worst fears are confirmed. The diagnosis is a "disc bulge" in the lumbar spine with "degenerative disc disease." The orthopedist discusses the surgery option with you, but you're not interested. The physical therapy continues.

As the pain goes on, you notice that you have developed "rituals" to manage your pain. Your morning routine might be awakening earlier than you would like because of the pain and taking pain medicine even before getting out of bed. The alarm finally goes off and you stand in a hot shower for quite some time to "loosen up" your back. You dress more slowly than you used to so as not to damage your back or possibly injure the "bulging disc" in your back. You drive to work using the lumbar pillow given you by the physical therapist. Concentrating on your work is difficult due to the pain, but you make it through another day. You head home looking forward to resting your back for the remainder of the evening.

As time goes on, you try other specialists to get more opinions about your pain. You see other orthopedists, neurologists, and a neurosurgeon. You try chiropractic manipulations, which feel good for a while, but the pain always returns. Acupuncture also helps for a while, but the pain returns when you try to increase your activity. Your orthopedist sends you to an anesthesiologist for a series of epidural nerve blocks (injections of anesthetic into the spine). The pain lingers.

You continue to protect your back. You have ceased doing most of the activities you used to enjoy because of the pain. Your sex life is so nonexistent that your spouse now jokingly refers to your waterbed as "the Dead Sea." You think, "What would happen if I moved the wrong way and that disc in my back ruptured?!" The thought is frightening and the pain continues. Sure, there are some good days, but these mostly involve sedentary activities. Golf, tennis, running, extended walking, extended sitting are not options with the pain. Long drives are definitely out. The pain controls your life.

Finally your tolerance level has reached a critical point. You decide you can't go on like this. You decide to have surgery. Surely that will cure the pain. After all, the MRI showed the problem and it just needs to be fixed.

Two weeks after surgery your pain does feel better. You have hope and encouragement after this initial relief. You decide to take it easy to be sure the pain relief continues. You begin to increase your activities slowly. The pain increases. You become more concerned. Three months after the operation the pain has returned to its original levels. You wonder, *Why did it return? What did I do?*

THE MULTIDISCIPLINARY APPROACH

Unfortunately this case example is not unusual, although it is quite preventable. Based on extensive research and clinical observations, several things have become clear about back pain. They are as follows:

- There are many different factors involved in the onset and continuation of back pain.

- Most back pain (80 to 90 percent) will resolve on its own within about four to eight weeks with or without treatment.

- If back pain does not resolve itself within four to eight weeks, or if it continues to recur, there are an overwhelming number of treatment options available to the sufferer.

- Most back-pain sufferers have no idea which treatments are effective or even the right questions to ask of their doctor. This opens them up to spending money on treatments that are ineffective or even make the back pain worse.

Given the above, where is a back-pain sufferer to turn for help? What can you do when the usual treatments of bed rest and anti-inflammatory medication administered by your family doctor do not work? The solution to this problem lies in what is now accepted as the only adequate approach to more complex back-pain problems: multidisciplinary evaluation and treatment.

The authors of this book practice in a setting where the multidisciplinary approach to back pain is used. In this approach the expertise of different specialists is combined to give the back-pain sufferer superior care. Spine centers such as ours are generally composed of the following specialists at a single location, which might also include state-of-the-art rehabilitation facilities:

- *Physiatrist:* a board-certified specialist in physical medicine and rehabilitation
- *Orthopedic surgeons* specializing in spinal disorders
- *Neurosurgeons* specializing in spinal disorders

- *Psychologists* with specialized training in pain evaluation and management
- *Anesthesiologists* who have specialized training in pain management and nerve blocks
- *Physical therapists* who have specialized training in spinal disorders
- *Occupational therapists* who have specialized training in job assessment and helping the patient return to work
- *Exercise physiologists* who have specialized training in spinal disorders and conditioning programs
- *Nurses*
- *Physicians' assistants*
- *Support staff* (includes physical-therapy assistants and technicians)
- *Availability and easy access to all latest technology and diagnostic testing, as well as consultant subspecialties*
- *Ph.D. researcher* to assess outcome data

In such a setting the highest level of expertise and quality care can be afforded to any back-pain sufferer, ranging from a simple sprained back to a complex spinal disorder. It is of course rare that a back-pain patient would see all of the above-listed specialists during the course of treatment. However, it is common that a person with a complex, chronic back-pain problem would be cared for simultaneously by multiple practitioners in the group who are in constant communication. As we shall see throughout this book, if problems of a complex nature are only treated by a single discipline, they are unlikely to improve.

The following includes descriptions of how patients are evaluated and treated when entering such a multidisciplinary spine center. This information will form the basis of learning how to get similar, high-quality treatment for your own back-pain problem.

The patient is often first evaluated with an extensive history and physical examination done by the physiatrist, a medical doctor specializing in physical medicine and rehabilitation. Although spine centers will include the involvement of different types of specialists, we have found physiatry particularly important in the treatment of back pain. The training of a physiatrist as it applies to a patient with back pain includes a four-year residency with extensive exposure to the nonsurgical aspects of orthopedics, neurology, rheumatology, general medicine, sports medicine, and rehabilitation medicine. The training also involves extensive exposure to physical therapy, exercise physiology, kinesiology, and pain psychology.

With an emphasis on painful disorders of the musculoskeletal system, most commonly back and neck pain, the physiatrist is uniquely skilled in the diagnosis of complex pain problems with an emphasis on nonsurgical treatment alternatives. Approaching patients from a "holistic" viewpoint, the physiatrist is able to consider physical factors, vocational needs, leisure activities and requirements, family and work situations, and other simultaneous medical problems as they pertain to the patient's back pain.

After completion of an extensive evaluation including the history and physical exam of approximately one hour (which is rarely seen in medicine these days), a decision is made regarding which other specialists in the group need to be involved in the treatment. It is at this crucial point that the team approach allows the expertise of various specialists to be utilized as needed. A few short case examples will clearly illustrate the advantages of such an approach. It should be mentioned that some of the terms and procedures discussed in the following examples may be foreign to you.

> **One purpose of this book is to make you an expert on obtaining the proper treatment for *your* back-pain problem.**

Once you have finished the book, the information in these examples will seem very familiar.

Example 1

Steve is a forty-year-old male computer programmer with a complaint of "on and off" back pain for two years. The pain has become persistent and progressively worse over the past three months. He has given up on his leisure activities of jogging and tennis and has had an increasingly difficult time getting through his workday because of back pain associated with prolonged sitting. He previously had four months of chiropractic manipulation, which gave him only short-term relief. He finds himself becoming increasingly irritable with his friends and family. He has become especially frustrated and angry in the past two months since his family doctor told him that his X rays are normal and there is nothing to do but live with the pain.

When he first came to the spine center a complete history and physical examination by the physiatrist revealed, among other things, that Steve had a sedentary job and a very high stress level. He had become increasingly deconditioned (weak) and had gained ten pounds in the past year since giving up running and tennis due to back pain. The examination revealed no signs of nerve damage or other underlying diseases that would require further diagnostic testing. He did show a fair degree of low-back muscle spasm and tenderness, poor posture, and weakened abdominal and trunk musculature, combined with a significantly high stress level. The patient was first reassured that his problem was benign (not life-threatening or dangerous) and reversible with no need for any further tests. A treatment plan of several components was outlined, requiring a team approach of specialists as follows:

- An aggressive rehabilitation program focusing on muscular reconditioning (strengthening) and trunk stabilization, to be carried out by both physical therapists and exercise physiologists. This treatment would sparingly utilize physical therapy modalities (e.g., hot and cold packs, ultrasound, massage) to reduce muscle spasm when needed as a complement to the aggressive reconditioning program.
- A stress and pain management program, performed by a

pain psychologist, with home techniques for relaxation and further insights as to the role of stress in perpetuating back pain.

- An occupational therapist to perform a job-site assessment and recommend modifications. This included addressing the patient's poor chair for back support and incorrect desk height and angles.
- Continued follow-up with the physiatrist, who would oversee and coordinate the team effort, along with providing continuing reassurance of the patient and assessing medication needs, if any, as the patient progresses.

Example 2

Carol is a thirty-two-year-old woman with six weeks of back pain radiating down the leg into the calf and foot, associated with some mild tingling and weakness. She works in sales and has had increasing difficulty with prolonged standing and walking, which is required in her job. She did have a CAT scan ordered by her general doctor, which showed evidence of an L4-5 disc herniation with nerve compression. An orthopedist had recommended that she have disc surgery, which was scheduled to be performed later that week. This woman was quite anxious about her upcoming surgery. Evidently her surgeon had implied that she might become paralyzed if she did not have the surgery. The evaluation and review of MRI films determined that the patient did indeed have a disc herniation with some evidence of nerve compression. The physiatrist concluded that the patient might well improve with an intensive course of conservative management, including epidural nerve blocks and aggressive physical therapy. It was also felt, however, that a second surgical consultation would be appropriate to help further reassure the patient and allay her anxiety about the conservative-approach decision.

The patient was seen that same day by the orthopedic spine surgeon, who evaluated her and extensively reassured her that further nonsurgical measures were appropriate. She was also educated about the natural history of disc herniations and that she had a very good possibility of avoiding surgery completely.

The surgeon reassured her that there was virtually no possibility of paralysis and no inherent danger in putting off the surgical option at this juncture.

The patient underwent a lumbar epidural blockade (injection of anesthetic into the back), from which she received significant pain relief. She subsequently started an aggressive program of lumbar stabilization, working with a physical therapist and exercise physiologist. The physiatrist began the patient on a course of anti-inflammatory medication, which was discontinued as the patient progressed through her program. Her symptoms completely resolved and she returned to her normal lifestyle.

Example 3
Jay is a forty-three-year-old male architect who has been on disability since his third spine surgery two years ago. He complains of persistent severe low back pain with radiation of pain down to his legs that awakens him every night. He is essentially homebound and uses high doses of codeine on a daily basis to help him cope with his pain. He has become severely depressed and has gained over thirty-five pounds over the past two years. His family life and financial situation have progressively deteriorated. He was told by his operating surgeon that nothing more can be done for his condition. He has attempted virtually every back-pain treatment available.

After initial evaluation of his case at the spine center, further diagnostic studies were ordered. Due to the chronic, complex nature of his pain problem, his case was presented at the weekly spine conference, in which all of the doctors discuss particularly difficult cases. In this meeting his diagnostic studies were reviewed by several orthopedic and neurosurgeons. It was determined that there was a small fragment of disc that continued to be compressing his nerve root at a level where his spine had become "unstable." This had caused a further narrowing of the nerve canal. A complex operation was planned that required the combined expertise of the neurosurgical and orthopedic spine surgeons. But prior to the surgery it was recommended that the patient complete a brief "preparation for surgery" treatment program to increase the likelihood of a good surgical response. This included decreasing his pain medications, teaching him pain-coping and relaxation techniques, and mild physical-therapy exercises to prepare him for the postoperative rehabilitation.

The operation was successfully completed, but the patient still needed an extensive course of multidisciplinary postoperative rehabilitation. This was done to address the multiple problems that had developed as a consequence of his chronic pain, including severe depression, excessive weight gain and muscular deconditioning, job loss, and finally, addiction to pain medication. His rehabilitation treatment required a team approach with the physiatrist, pain psychologist, physical therapists, exercise physiologists, occupational therapist, and vocational counselors, along with postoperative follow-up by the orthopedic and neurosurgical spine specialists. Four months after the operation the patient's pain was at minimal levels and he was off all pain medications. In addition, he was interviewing for jobs and was no longer depressed.

Example 4

Patty is a thirty-one-year-old secretary with complaints of pain throughout her back, as well as occasional neck and shoulder pain and intermittent headaches. She also complains of increasing fatigue, difficulty sleeping, and occasional tingling in her hands and feet. She had been under tremendous job stress because she had been having problems with a new supervisor over the past year. Her physical examination was within normal limits, except for multiple areas of muscle tenderness throughout her body. This pattern is characteristically found in what has been termed tension myalgia syndrome or stress-related back pain.

The patient was educated and reassured about the benign nature of her pain syndrome, which is known to be stress-related. In this condition stress or emotional factors are thought to be primary in the initiation and maintenance of the back-pain problem. This would be similar to other types of stress-related conditions, such as tension headaches, stomachaches, and irritable bowel syndrome, among others. Stress-related back pain commonly results in painful spasms to the neck and back muscles as well as fatigue and a feeling of generalized weakness.

She was started on an aggressive exercise program with the exercise physiologists, along with a biofeedback stress-management program, as directed by the pain psychologist. She had a full resolution of her symptoms and returned to normal function in three weeks.

Example 5

Robert is a seventy-four-year-old self-employed man who had continued to manage his own business full-time until seven months prior to his initial visit. He had been experiencing increasing back and leg pain, which was becoming more disabling. As a result he had decreased his workload to part-time, had stopped his exercise routine, and had cut down on most of his socializing. He was spending much of his time at home either on the couch or in bed and he was experiencing increasing depression as a result of his pain.

The initial evaluation revealed degenerative disc disease (related to aging) as well as lumbar spinal stenosis (a narrowing of the spinal canal in the lumbar region of the spine). It appeared that the process had been going on for many years, but the patient had only recently noticed the disabling symptoms. This condition is seen commonly in elderly persons and it was having a profound impact on Robert.

The physical findings suggested the patient would respond to a rehabilitation program involving a number of components. First he was started on a special physical-therapy program (pelvic tilt and flexion exercises) to help decrease the stenosis and to recondition his body. A brief trial of anti-inflammatory medicines was also done. Lastly the patient worked with the physician and the psychologist to develop realistic expectations about his functional status and to help resolve the depression that had occurred. The patient was clearly experiencing a grief reaction (or depression) over not being able to perform at his previous level. In response to this he had virtually given up on all activities. This emotional state had significantly increased his pain and disability.

A more detailed examination of the above cases will demonstrate the value of a multidisciplinary approach. In the first case the patient required simultaneous attention to the multiple factors contributing to his problem. This included modifications of his work environment along with an aggressive rehabilitation program. Although the patient's problems were not particularly complex, he had been unable to find a solution previously by seeing a variety of individual doctors. This illustrates an important aspect of multidisciplinary treatment for back pain. Patients will often try various treatment approaches (e.g., physical therapy, medications, injections, manipulations) one at a time. The theory is that if one doesn't work, then try another. In multidisciplinary treatment there is something very powerful in completing all appropriate treatments *simultaneously in a coordinated fashion.* This issue will be addressed repeatedly throughout this book.

In example 2 the patient was saved from undergoing an unnecessary spine surgery for a herniated disc. As we commonly see, her condition responded quite well to aggressive conservative management with a team approach. Although the physiatrist was quite confident that the approach would be effective, an orthopedic spine surgeon further assured the patient that a surgical intervention was not necessary nor was paralysis likely. After the spine surgeon explained to the patient that only a very small minority of orthopedists are experts in both surgical and nonsurgical management of herniated discs, she was able to understand that her previous orthopedist could not offer a nonsurgical approach, since surgery is the focus of his practice. He did not have a team of specialists to assist him in the care of nonsurgical patients or in postoperative rehabilitation of his surgical patients. This is of critical importance because even when a back surgery is needed, it is only part of the solution. Surgical outcomes are greatly improved with proper preoperative and postoperative rehabilitation.

In example 3 we saw a spinal problem of a very complex nature involving multiple failed surgeries. The appropriate surgical intervention clearly required a high level of surgical expertise in the area of spine surgery rarely found in the fields of orthopedic and neurosurgery in a general sense. It should be noted that a recommendation for further surgery in a case of this nature is also extremely rare and is based on very specific criteria. A combined surgical approach was necessary in conjunction with pre- and post-operative team treatment. This multidisciplinary team approach was the only way of solving this man's problems. In fact utilizing this approach in the first place might have helped the patient avoid the three failed spine surgeries altogether!

In example 4 we saw a very prevalent condition that is known as tension myalgia syndrome or stress-related back pain. The condition will be fully discussed in later chapters. Unfortunately this problem is rarely recognized by the majority of health care specialists who evaluate and treat patients with back problems. Being aware of the multiple factors that can cause and maintain back pain will help ensure that such a diagnosis is not overlooked.

In example 5 we saw a common clinical picture of back pain in the elderly. The patient had been highly functional until the conditions of his degenerative disc disease and spinal stenosis became symptomatic. This resulted in a virtual and complete deterioration in physical and emotional functioning. In the treatment it was important to address the physical rehabilitation as well as the grief reaction, fear of aging, and depression. Part of this treatment was to help the patient accept the very real limitations that would be caused by the lumbar stenosis while also achieving the highest level of functioning (physically and socially) possible. Not addressing all of these issues simultaneously would have resulted in the patient's continued disability and depression.

The advantages of a multidisciplinary approach become quite clear in reviewing the above examples. Although many patients with back problems may do well with an individual practitioner, no one individual specialist can adequately treat many of the difficult back-pain problems and associated features. The future will certainly see an increasing number of multidisciplinary spine centers handling patients with back pain at the highest level of expertise. However, the availability of these centers remains quite limited at present. Nevertheless the person with back pain and no access to such a center does not need to continue to suffer without receiving quality care. This book will show you how to get the benefits of a multidisciplinary treatment center even if one is not available in your community.

ABOUT THIS BOOK

This book was written to give you a complete approach to your back-pain problem. The following key issues will be addressed:

- **How to understand traditional back-pain diagnoses**
  Having accurate information about the diagnoses you will be confronted with is essential for you to avoid the fear that often comes with these labels. This understanding will also help you see why the multidisciplinary aggressive-physical-conditioning approach, while paying attention to emotional factors, is the answer to most back pain.

- **How to avoid inappropriate and possibly harmful treatments**
  Much of the information presented will educate you about the most common evaluations and treatments for back pain. This will help you obtain the proper treatment and steer clear of inappropriate and often harmful treatments. We find that educating patients about what treatments they *should not* do helps build the necessary foundation for them to accept wholeheartedly what treatments they *should do*.

- **The need to engage in physical and mental reconditioning**
  The cornerstone of our approach is physical conditioning

while paying attention to any factors that may be preventing a full recovery. This reconditioning is done using a specialized approach while keeping the fear of pain under control.

- **The need to pay attention to emotions and attitudes**
  This is probably to most ignored and misunderstood area in the treatment of back pain while possibly being the most important. Throughout the book each topic will be discussed within the context of mind-body issues. Finally, the entire last section focuses exclusively on how attitudes and emotions can affect your back pain and how to address these issues as part of getting better.

HOW TO USE THIS BOOK

The goal of this book is to give you the tools necessary to play an active role in obtaining multidisciplinary treatment for your back pain within your community. This will usually involve a working partnership with your physician to obtain the appropriate care for your individual problem. More specifically this book will enable you to discuss and consider a variety of diagnostic and therapeutic options with your doctor. After such discussions you and your doctor can assemble the necessary treatment team using the principles of a multidisciplinary spine center.

The information in this book will give you the newest knowledge about back pain and put you on the road to relief from your suffering.

CHAPTER 2

WORKING WITH YOUR DOCTOR

As we will discuss extensively in other chapters, back pain affects more than 75 percent of the population at some time during their lifetime. Back pain is second only to the common cold as a reason for visits to the doctor, and second only to childbirth as a reason for hospitalization. People with back pain will consult a variety of health care professionals and paraprofessionals in search of relief. To list all of these providers would be exhaustive, but the common ones include the family doctor, a general practitioner or internist, an orthopedist or neurosurgeon. Other practitioners might include chiropractors, osteopaths, acupuncturists, and massage therapists, just to name a few.

In managing your back pain it is important to understand the type of doctors who treat back pain, as well as analyzing the relationship you have with your doctor. It is important to enter into a treating relationship with your doctor feeling that you are an equal partner and taking an equal amount of responsibility for your improvement. Patients who enter into the relationship feeling that the doctor is going to "fix" their back pain are at an increased risk for disappointment.

As we will discuss in chapter 3, "Myths About Back Pain," ambiguity and confusion are common in the area of back-pain diagnosis and treatment. Patients often go to the doctor believing that the criteria for diagnoses are specific and the treatment approaches are proven effective. This could not be farther from the truth.

It has been estimated that 80 percent or more of back-pain problems are never specifically diagnosed and that 90 percent of back pain will resolve on its own with or without treatment.

These findings provide fertile ground for professionals claiming that it was "their" treatment that worked when in fact the pain would have gone away regardless. Still, many doctors who treat back pain will attempt to provide a reasonable-sounding explanation for the pain simply to fulfill their patient's need for a diagnosis. Doing this gives the patient the sense that the doctor knows what he or she is doing. Then, when the pain decreases, the doctor (or other practitioner) takes credit. This can lead to a variety of unnecessary treatments and in some cases cause more harm than good.

This chapter will discuss how to have a safe and effective relationship with your doctor. First we will discuss some of the various professionals who treat back pain. We will also discuss how to become an informed and smart consumer in obtaining treatment for your back-pain problem. This section will include various questions to ask your doctor or treating practitioner to ensure that you are fully informed regarding his or her approach. Finally we will discuss the importance of the relationship between you and your treating professional(s) and provide you with a self-assessment approach to make this relationship the best it can be.

DOCTORS WHO WORK WITH BACK PAIN

There are a variety of professionals who deal with back pain. It is beyond the scope of this book to list all of the treating professionals who manage back-pain problems. Instead we will briefly discuss the most common disciplines that treat back pain and give you some guidelines for making decisions regarding treatment approaches.

Organization of the Medical Community

Entering the medical culture can be a scary and confusing excursion. The medical community has its own organization, language, and customs. This book will serve as a map to help you chart a positive course.

It is important to understand how the medical community is arranged in terms of *levels* of specialization. The first level is your family doctor or general practitioner, who handles a variety of medical problems. These doctors should have a good understanding of all aspects of medicine and often act as *coordinators* or *managers* of your treatment.

The second level of doctors who treat back pain are the *specialists*. This might include such medical specialties as orthopedics, neurology, neurosurgery, and physiatry (a physical-medicine doctor). We will discuss more about these specialists later in this chapter.

The third level of treating doctors would include the *subspecialist*. These are orthopedists, neurosurgeons, and physiatrists who have further specialized training specifically in spine disorders and back pain.

Therefore in traditional medical practice there are three levels of treating doctors through which you might proceed. The same type of levels of specialization might also occur in alternative health care models, including chiropractic and osteopathy.

The following types of doctors are the most common ones people see for back pain. This list is by no means complete, but it will give you a general idea of what type of practitioners commonly treat back-pain problems.

General Practitioners, Internal Medicine, and Family Practice Physicians

These primary health care professionals are usually the ones that are consulted first for any type of medical problem, including back pain. They are equipped to handle a variety of medical problems, and often they are comfortable and confident treating back-pain problems. It is likely that these professionals will actually be treating more back-pain problems in the future

21

as the use of specialists is discouraged under health care reform and the financial pressures of managed care. Several think-tank panels have recommended that general practitioners be educated and equipped to handle most straightforward back-pain problems. In working with your family doctor or internist, it is important to know whether he or she is comfortable treating a back-pain problem. These doctors will usually make sure there is nothing seriously wrong with your spine and will then treat you during the acute phase (the first six to eight weeks). If other symptoms occur, or the pain lingers, you may be referred to a specialist.

Orthopedists, Neurosurgeons, and Physiatrists

Doctors in orthopedics, neurosurgery, and physiatry are the specialists most likely to receive referrals for back pain. As discussed above, although these are specialty areas, they may not have a primary focus on spinal disorders and back pain. These specialties require a residency after general medical or surgical training, as well as a board certification examination. Orthopedics and neurosurgery are disciplines of medicine with which most people are familiar. Physiatrists are medical doctors with special training in physical medicine, rehabilitation, and musculoskeletal (the muscles and bones) disorders. They use nonsurgical, conservative treatment approaches for musculoskeletal and other medical problems, including back pain.

If you are referred to one of these specialists, confirm that the doctor has competency in treating back pain and is familiar with a conservative approach. Orthopedists and neurosurgeons do a surgical residency and are primarily trained in surgical approaches to medical problems. Although many are comfortable with a conservative approach to back pain, many are not. This issue is discussed further in the chapter on spine surgery.

The Subspecialties

Any of the above specialties can further specialize in the area of spinal disorders and back pain. This would include advanced training in the area of spinal disorders and back pain, as well as having a medical practice that primarily focuses on that area. Although orthopedists, neurosurgeons, and physiatry are probably the most common disciplines that would subspecialize in spinal disorders, other areas of medicine might also focus on back pain.

QUESTIONS TO ASK YOUR DOCTOR

The book *Smart Questions to Ask Your Doctor* outlines how to obtain information about selecting a doctor, as well as diagnostic and treatment approaches. The following lists combine general issues from that book along with many of our own questions, which apply specifically to back-pain problems. Using these questions in finding a treating professional for your back-pain problem will help you get the highest quality of care and avoid such things as unnecessary and harmful treatments. We should reiterate that most back-pain problems will not require the care of either a specialist or a subspecialist. The majority of acute back-pain problems can be safely managed by a person's family doctor. *In fact as we will discuss throughout this book, many primary practitioners and specialists will provide treatments that are actually more harmful than obtaining no treatment at all.*

- **What is your degree?**
  It is important to determine what professional degree the treating practitioner holds. There are a variety of professionals who go by the term *doctor* who are not medical physicians. Groups that are referred to as "Doctor" but do not have medical training might include such degrees as a Ph.D. (e.g., in exercise physiology, physical therapy and nursing), D.C. (Doctor of Chiropractic), D.O. (Doctor of Osteopathy), and a variety of "doctorates" in alternative medicine practice.

- **Where did you do your training?**
  You should have an understanding of where your doctor

did his or her training in terms of both medical school education and internship and residency.

- **Are you a board-certified specialist?**
  In medicine, board certification in a specialty is done by completing a multiyear residency and passing a national board-certification examination. Specialists, such as orthopedists, neurosurgeons, and physiatrists, must obtain specialized training and demonstrate excellence in their specialty area. You should inquire as to where your doctor did his or her residency and when he or she passed the specialty board-certification examination.

  It is important to distinguish between the terms *board-eligible* and *board-certified.* "Board-eligible" simply means that the doctor has completed the required training, but has not yet passed the examination.

  Board certification is also done in areas other than medicine. Most professional groups have constructed a certification process. For instance there is board certification for chiropractors, osteopaths, psychologists, and physical therapists, as well as for many other disciplines. Virtually any health care practitioner can train to be a specialist in areas beyond general practice.

  In areas other than medicine be sure to ask how the board certification was completed. Currently there are many so-called board-certification credentials that can be obtained simply by filling out a form and sending it in with an appropriate amount of "dues" payment. This can be misleading to the general public, who assume that the board certification actually documents a higher level of specialized training.

- **What medical and professional societies do you belong to?**
  Assessing the types of medical and/or professional societies that your doctor belongs to can give you an idea of his or her treatment focus. For instance there are the general medical and professional societies relevant to each discipline. Beyond that there are a number of specialized soci-

eties in the area of spinal disorders and back-pain problems, including the following:

American Back Society
Society for the Study of the Lumbar Spine
North American Spine Society
International Association for the Study of Pain
American Pain Society

Membership in these societies, as well as others not listed, usually indicates that the health care professional is obtaining continuing education in the area of spinal problems and back pain.

- **How long have you practiced in this area?**
Finding a doctor who has had a number of years practicing in the community can help in terms of treatment "networking." Although all doctors have to start out new in practice at some point, a doctor at a well-established practice is more likely to have a good understanding of the community resources available. Examples of this include

1. Other specialists in the community who might be utilized during the course of your back-pain treatment
2. Community resources that might be helpful for continued treatment of your back pain, such as community exercise programs and swimming pool facilities
3. Vocational rehabilitation assistance and training programs

- **Have you had special training in treating back-pain problems?**
This would involve addressing the subspecialty issue. Health care professionals may specialize beyond general training, but have no subspecialty experience with spinal disorders or back-pain problems. Subspecialization in this

area would include further training, as well as a practice that is primarily limited to spine and back pain. Subspecialization can be somewhat rare in smaller communities and is most often always available through university medical schools.

• **Are you comfortable treating back pain using a conservative approach?**
You need to find out if your treating doctor is comfortable and competent using a conservative approach to back pain. This question especially needs to be asked of specialists who are trained primarily as surgeons. As we discuss in chapter 12, almost all surgery on the spine is elective. This means that the conservative approach is primary.

• **What percentage of your practice deals with back-pain problems?**
This question is generally asked of specialists and can give you a good idea of how much experience the treating doctor has in back-pain problems. This information can usually be obtained from the office manager. Going to a doctor who has specialized in spinal disorders would automatically ensure that his practice is primarily made up of this patient population group.

You can obtain much of the needed information simply by requesting a copy of the doctor's curriculum vitae or résumé. Most offices will have this on file and should be more than willing to provide you with this information prior to even scheduling your first appointment. You can scan the vitae and determine the answers to many of the preceding questions.

Obtaining answers to these questions should be done in a realistic fashion. It is unrealistic to expect that a doctor will take the time to answer all of them prior to scheduling the initial appointment or even as part of the initial appointment; therefore obtain all the information you can from the doctor's résumé and then ask any remaining questions.

CHIROPRACTORS AND OSTEOPATHS

Many people with back pain are treated by chiropractors and osteopaths either primarily or in addition to medical care. This section will discuss how to approach chiropractic care in an informed manner, similar to what was discussed above in the area of medicine. Many of the questions outlined above can be used if you decide to seek chiropractic care for your back pain. Beyond these there are also special concerns to take into account when obtaining this type of treatment.

Chiropractors will generally approach the treatment of back pain through the use of spinal manipulation, modalities (hot packs, ultrasound, massage), and mild exercise. Although other disciplines will also use spinal manipulation, this is the mainstay of chiropractic practice. Although research in the area of spinal manipulation for treating back pain is minimal, there are some studies that suggest that appropriate use of spinal manipulation can help. The research generally concludes that spinal manipulation is most likely to be useful in back pain that is less than three weeks in duration and where there is no damage to the spinal nerves going to the legs. It does appear that although this type of back pain will usually remit on its own, spinal manipulation appears to accelerate the normal course of recovery.

If you are obtaining chiropractic care for back pain, or if it has been suggested, you should take into account the following questions and issues.*

- **See your physician first.**
  You should have a medical doctor evaluate your back pain prior to obtaining chiropractic care. This is essential to rule out serious causes of back pain, which are discussed later in this book. Although these are extremely rare, they do occur. Also your medical doctor can determine

---

* These questions have been adapted from an article on chiropractic practice in *Consumer Reports,* June 1994.

whether chiropractic care would be a safe treatment for you. Spinal manipulation is not recommended if you have a fracture, rheumatoid arthritis, severe osteoporosis, bleeding disorders, or infection or inflammation of the spine.

- **Get a referral from a reliable source.**
  The primary societies for chiropractors are the National Association for Chiropractic Medicine and the Orthopedic Manipulation Society International, both of which maintain referral lists of chiropractors. You might also get referrals from family and friends who have had positive treatment experiences. When getting referrals from nonprofessionals who have had treatment, it is useful to ask about the nature of the treatment provided (number of sessions, etc.) and the outcome.

- **Ask questions.**
  Many of the questions recommended for medical specialties can also be used in working with a chiropractor. Other specific questions include the following:

  - **Do you treat primarily musculoskeletal problems?**
  - **Will you work with my medical doctor?**
  - **Will you recommend exercises and other things I can do at home?**
  - **Will you tell me how long and how often I should expect to be treated?**

  Research has indicated that a patient with back pain should be feeling better and showing signs of improvement within nine to twelve sessions of manipulation.

- **Watch out for the warning signs of poor practice.**
  You should be concerned if the chiropractor does any of the following:
  1. Takes full spine or repeated X rays.
  2. Fails to do a complete history and clinical examination prior to beginning treatment.

3. Claims the treatment will improve immune function or cure disease.
4. Offers a variety of "vitamin cures" or "homeopathic" remedies.
5. Tries to get other family members to begin treatment.
6. Wants you to sign a contract for long-term care.
7. Promises to prevent disease through regular checkups or manipulation. This would also apply to promising to prevent back pain through regular manipulations, as there is absolutely no research to support this claim.
8. Implies that chiropractic can be viewed as a primary health care modality.

Just as we suggested in investigating a medical specialist, you may want to ask for a chiropractor's or osteopath's vitae/résumé.

YOUR RELATIONSHIP WITH YOUR DOCTOR

Your relationship with your doctor or other health care professional treating your back-pain problem is extremely important. Often your expectations will not match the expectations of your doctor, and this can become a significant blockade to good treatment. For instance you may expect that your doctor will simply diagnose the problem and then "do something to you" to get rid of it. This type of passivity on a patient's part in the treatment of back pain can have disastrous results. Back pain is best treated when both the patient and the doctor have an active role in solving your back-pain problem. Many patients are reluctant to take such a role, as it requires an increased level of assertiveness and responsibility. In addition many doctors are uncomfortable with patients who want to be fully involved in their treatment. If you do not take an active role, you are at increased risk for a variety of unnecessary treatments, such as passive physical therapy that goes on too long, inappropriate medicines, unnecessary surgery, and other treatments that are not beneficial.

In order to assess the relationship between a doctor and patient, the Trust in Physician Scale (TPS) was developed. This measure was developed by Dr. Lynda Anderson to assess a patient's trust in his or her physician. We have modified the TPS for use with doctors treating back pain.

TPS

Each item below is a statement with which you may agree or disagree. Beside each statement is a scale that ranges from strongly agree (1) to strongly disagree (5). For each item circle the number that represents the extent to which you agree or disagree with the statement.

Make sure that you answer every item and that you circle only one number per item. It is important that you respond according to what you actually believe and not according to what you feel you should believe.

> **1 = Strongly agree**   **4 = Disagree**
> **2 = Agree**   **5 = Strongly disagree**
> **3 = Neutral**

1. I doubt that my doctor really cares about me as a person. **1 2 3 4 5**
2. My doctor is usually considerate of my needs and puts them first. **1 2 3 4 5**
3. I trust my doctor so much, I will always follow her or his advice regarding my back pain. **1 2 3 4 5**
4. If my doctor tells me something is so, then it must be true. **1 2 3 4 5**
5. I sometimes mistrust my doctor's opinion about my back pain and would like a second one. **1 2 3 4 5**
6. I trust my doctor's judgments about my medical care for my back pain. **1 2 3 4 5**
7. I feel my doctor does not do everything he or she should for my back pain. **1 2 3 4 5**
8. I trust my doctor to put my medical needs above all other considerations when treating my back pain. **1 2 3 4 5**
9. My doctor is a real expert in taking care of back-pain problems like mine. **1 2 3 4 5**

(continued on next page)

TPS *(continued)*

10. I trust my doctor to tell me if a mistake was made about my treatment. **1 2 3 4 5**
11. I sometimes worry that my doctor may not keep the information we discuss totally private. **1 2 3 4 5**

To score the TPS, items 1, 5, 7, and 11 are "reverse scored." For those items you score the exact opposite of what you marked. For instance if you circled a "1," that would count as "5"; if you circled a "2," that would count as "4"; and if you circled a "3," that would count as "3." All other items are simply scored at the number value that you marked. Score each question and add the total number of items after reverse scoring items 1, 5, 7, and 11. The higher score reflects more trust in your treating professional. In the research sample studied, averages ranged from 48 to approximately 57.

Source: Trust in Physician Scale © 1990. Used by permission of Dr. Lynda A. Anderson, School of Public Health, University of Michigan, Ann Arbor, MI.

A good, trusting relationship with your doctor is very important in the successful outcome of your treatment. Even so, we must also emphasize that "blind trust" is not a healthy way to approach treatment for your back-pain problem. You should have a high level of trust in your treating professional while also feeling comfortable to be skeptical of any recommendations. You should be able to question your doctor as to the reasons for the recommendations and the anticipated results. Your doctor should also be comfortable with you obtaining a second, or even third, opinion at any time. This issue is discussed further in other chapters.

CHAPTER 3

MYTHS ABOUT BACK PAIN

This chapter will cover a great number of the common myths about back pain. These myths are held by doctors as well as laypeople. First we will present a Back Pain IQ Test so that you can assess your current understanding of back pain. Once you have completed reading this chapter, return to the Back Pain IQ Test and see how you would answer differently.

TESTING YOUR BACK PAIN IQ

Having a good understanding of the true nature of back pain is essential to getting proper care, avoiding unnecessary and often dangerous procedures, and relieving suffering. The following questions will test your knowledge of back pain. As we have found in working with many people with back pain, you will find the results very surprising!

	TRUE	FALSE
• If you have back pain, there is definitely something injuring your back.	___	___
• Bed rest is the best thing for back pain.	___	___
• The back is a relatively weak structure that is prone to injury.	___	___
• Back-pain problems and disability due to back pain are worse in third-world countries because they don't have modern treatment approaches.	___	___
• The best principle to follow for back pain is always to "let pain be your guide."	___	___
• "Pain is pain," no matter how you think or feel about it.	___	___

(continued on next page)

TESTING YOUR BACK PAIN IQ *(continued)*	TRUE	FALSE
• The older you get, the more back pain you will have.	____	____
• A herniated disc in your back requires surgery to correct the problem.	____	____
• Back pain is very uncommon.	____	____
• Doctors can almost always find the cause of back pain.	____	____
• If you are physically fit, you are less likely to have back pain.	____	____
• Treatments commonly used to treat back pain are the most effective.	____	____
• The amount of pain you feel is directly related to the damage in your back.	____	____
• Doctors have a good understanding of most back-pain ailments.	____	____
• Chronic back pain (more than six months) means your back is severely damaged.	____	____
• Once you hurt your back, it will never be the same.	____	____

MYTHS ABOUT BACK PAIN

There are many common misconceptions about back pain held by both laypeople, patients, and doctors. In fact after reading this book you may very well know more of the current facts about back pain than your doctor. As we discussed in the first chapter, these commonly held misbeliefs lead to unnecessary treatments and surgery. As Dr. Stan Herring of the University of Washington has stated, "As it is, by and large, the medical community overreacts to back ailments. Back problems are overmedicated, overrested, and overoperated." These unnecessary practices, based largely on the following medical myths, are not only expensive but also can have disastrous consequences for the person with back pain. If you have experienced back pain and the typical treatments, then you may be well aware of these consequences. We have treated countless people with back pain who have become terrified of their pain, in good part, as a result of their previous treatments. This fear is perpetuated by incorrect information and treatment approaches. As we shall see, statements such as "You need to be careful not to reinjure your back," "Let the pain be your guide," and "You have a bulging disc in your spine along with degenerative disc disease; you have the spine of an eighty-year-old" all serve to increase confusion and fear. They can also lead to unnecessary treatment, emotional distress, and worsened pain!

The frustrating part of this process is that there is no need for the level of suffering that most people with back pain experience. The following medical myths will help you understand just how much incorrect information exists in the area of back pain and also help ease some of the common fears about the condition.

This chapter serves as a general overview of the entire book by portraying the myths established by the latest research discussed in chapter 1. Subsequent chapters will explore these myths in more detail and give the newest knowledge about back pain and back-pain treatment.

Myth 1: If I have back pain, there must be something damaging my back.

Truth: There are many known and well-understood structural causes of back pain, which will be covered in this book. However, in the great majority of back-pain cases there is no agreed-upon structural cause. In fact Dr. Stanley Bigos of the University of Washington Medical School has estimated that the medical community only specifically understands about 12 percent of back ailments that are treated. The pain may be generated by one of several structures, with medical experts commonly offering different opinions. The specific cause remains unknown in the great majority of cases, especially in chronic back pain, when multiple factors often come into play. It has been estimated that even with the best medical evaluation, in 85 percent of back-pain cases a definite diagnosis as to the cause of the pain is not found. Despite the lack of a clear structural cause or the ability to pinpoint a diagnosis, the prognosis remains excellent in most cases of back pain. In fact 80 to 90 percent of back-pain episodes resolve within twelve weeks, and some studies suggest this will occur with or without formal treatment.

Myth 2: The back is a delicate structure that is easily injured.

Truth: The back is actually a very strong structure and can withstand tremendous forces without injury when the surrounding musculature is properly conditioned. This muscular conditioning involves strength, flexibility, and endurance. Proper body mechanics and posture (e.g., how you move your body when doing such things as picking up objects, standing, and sitting) further reduces the risk of back injury along with reducing the work required for a specific task. Proper conditioning techniques and body mechanics will be discussed in greater detail in later chapters.

Myth 3: As one gets older, the spine gets weaker and back pain gets worse.

Truth: Several studies have actually shown that the prevalence of back pain *decreases* in the latter decades, with the peak incidence from thirty-five to fifty-five years of age. Although back pain doesn't necessarily get worse as one gets older, we do know that the spine continues to degenerate to some degree throughout our lives. This is a normal part of the aging process. Although these degenerative changes of the spine continue to progress, as is often recognized on radiographic studies, there is no consistent corresponding increase in the degree of back pain. In fact we very often see severely degenerative spinal changes in elderly patients without evidence of back pain. Furthermore one is never too old to properly condition and strengthen one's back.

The traditional medical approach is to view these degenerative changes as abnormal and pathologic ("degenerative disc disease") and to target them as the reason for any back pain.

This of course can lead to unnecessary treatment and an attempt to "fix" the problem. We need to accept these changes in our spines as we accept all other changes associated with aging.

Myth 4: The best thing for back pain is rest.

Truth: Rest is often helpful for acute back pain when used for approximately three days. A study published in the *New England Journal of Medicine* by Dr. Richard Deyo found two to three days of bed rest to be beneficial for acute back pain in most cases. However, it is very well known that prolonged bed rest, as was and still is commonly employed by physicians, is not only not helpful but often harmful. Prolonged bed rest (which we can consider greater than five days) is associated with an increase of muscle deconditioning, which can have very debilitating effects. The deconditioning worsens over time, which can perpetuate a chronic pain syndrome. Unfortunately many individuals as well as health care professionals are unaware of these facts and continue to utilize long-term bed rest for symptomatic relief, unnecessarily prolonging their disability. However, in rare cases, such as unstable spinal fracture, long-term bed rest may be required under the strict guidance of a medical spine specialist.

As far as the rationale for bed rest, there are two widely accepted thoughts. First is that bed rest minimizes the pressure on the discs in the spine, which are the "cushions" in between each of the vertebrae (the bones in your spine). Second is that bed rest reduces any mechanical stresses that might be irritating pain receptors. The problem with this reasoning is that it assumes there is something "broken" in the back that needs to be rested. As we have discussed, this is rarely the case.

There are other problems with this rationale of bed rest. Studies have shown that if you are in bed resting on your back, rolling on your side will raise the pressure on your discs up to 75 percent of the total pressure from when you are standing! Also many people will get bed rest for back pain while propping themselves up with pillows to watch TV or read. This position actually causes more pressure on the disc than if you are standing. The argument against long-term bed rest was confirmed in the Deyo study, which compared two days and seven days of bed rest and found that patients in the former group returned to work 45 percent sooner than the seven-day group.

There are possible serious consequences of prolonged bed rest, although it is still widely prescribed and practiced. These include (a) perception of a severe illness and perpetuation of a sickness role (even a heart attack does not require a week of strict bed rest); (b) economic losses; (c) muscle weakening and atrophy at an astounding rate of 1 to 1.5 percent per day; (d) cardiopulmonary deconditioning (15 percent in ten days); (e) bone mineral loss; and (f) deep venous thrombosis and thromboembolism.

In summary, short-term bed rest up to two to three days has proven efficacious in almost all cases of low back pain. Prolonged bed rest is not indicated for virtually all cases of back pain and will not help it. The prolonged bed rest will also have potential negative side effects, which can actually extend the length of the pain.

Myth 5: Once you have back pain, you must be very careful to protect your back.

Truth: Many people often overprotect their backs. Obsessively trying to protect and guard your back stems from thinking of your spine as weak, fragile, and easily injured, which we have seen is just not true. Too much bed rest is one way in which people overprotect their backs. However, protecting one's back even without bed rest might present several complications. After an episode of back pain many individuals make the switch from a very active lifestyle including many physical and sporting activities to an extremely sedentary one. This is done in an effort to protect themselves from further injury, although this inactivity frequently leads to deconditioning and worsening of their symptoms.

Protecting your back should only go as far as incorporating proper body mechanics and properly conditioning the muscles that are utilized in most activities. There are certain exceptions to this, such as spinal instability, fractures of several types that do require multiple restrictions upon the patient. However, in the majority of individuals with back pain it is not necessary to be overprotective. Patients often have a tendency to be obsessive about their posture and body mechanics to the point of developing extremely unnatural and often restrictive movements. This is based more on fear than on medical rationale. Experiencing back pain does not mean one needs to stop bending, twisting, and lifting.

Myth 6: The only successful treatment for a herniated disc is surgery.

Truth: Actually surgery is only indicated for a minority of patients with herniated discs. A study published by Dr. Jeffrey Saal in the journal *Spine* found 92 percent of patients with documented disc herniations to recover adequately with non-surgical conservative management. Many of the patients in this study had large herniated discs that compressed nerve roots and they still managed to avoid a surgical option. Another study looked at patients with disc herniations treated surgically and nonsurgically and found no difference after five years. In some cases there may be a decrease in the period of disability in an appropriate surgery group.

It is becoming clearer that there is a tremendously high incidence (up to 35 percent) of herniated discs in people without back or leg pain. In other words if we randomly selected one hundred individuals off the street without back pain, we would find evidence of a herniated disc in up to thirty-five of those individuals!

We also often see the symptoms associated with disc herniation and nerve compression resolve spontaneously as the disc shrinks. A recent study utilizing CT scan to observe disc herniations demonstrated radiologically that large herniated discs often shrink on their own after six months. There are, however, certain disc herniations that can cause progressive neurologic loss and do require surgery to avoid potential permanent neurologic loss. This determination, however, should only be made by a spine specialist who is aware of nonsurgical treatment options, which are often a reasonable alternative.

Myth 7: You should let the pain be your guide in managing your back pain.

Truth: In the vast majority of cases of chronic back pain, this is not true. Letting pain be one's guide is often based on the often-incorrect premise that pain is equated with further injury. This may hold true for acute back pain, which we can arbitrarily define as lasting up to one month. For subacute back pain, which we can define as lasting from two to six months, this statement is somewhat true. However, in chronic back pain, greater than six months, pain should rarely be the guide except in very specific diagnoses as determined by a spine specialist (including spinal instability, symptomatic disc herniations, etc.).

It is very common to see individuals with chronic benign back pain unnecessarily limit their lifestyles by letting pain be their guide. Most respected academic chronic pain centers in fact take just the opposite approach. They focus on activity and functional restoration in spite of one's pain, attempting to recondition the body and return the individual to an active lifestyle. Furthermore, in chronic back pain the pain itself is often a consequence of other factors having little to do with the patient's back, as we will discuss in greater detail later.

Myth 8: My father or mother have back pain and so will I.

Truth: Back pain is usually not hereditary. There is no genetic predisposition to back pain shown in most cases and there is virtually no reason to conclude that just because your parents had back pain, then you will suffer as well.

Myth 9: Back pain is very uncommon.

Truth: Back pain is actually extremely common, affecting up to 80 percent of the population at some point in their lifetime.

It is the leading cause of disabilities in males under forty-five years of age and represents a $50 billion problem annually. It is the second most frequent reason for a visit to the doctor, the fifth most common cause for hospitalization, and the third highest reason for surgical procedures. Approximately 1 percent of the U.S. population is chronically disabled due to back pain, and another 1 percent are temporarily disabled. Combined, this represents over five million people. We firmly believe that much of this treatment and disability is unnecessary and in good part influenced by our cultural and individual attitudes toward back pain.

Myth 10: Health professionals have a good understanding of how to treat back pain.

Truth: Unfortunately there is much disagreement among health practitioners as to the best treatment approaches for individuals with back pain. In fact there is probably less standardization in the diagnosis and treatment of back pain than of any other medical ailment. Of course there are certain specific cases where there is a consensus among medical professionals as to the proper treatment. These diagnoses (tumors, infections, fractures, etc.) only represent a minority, while the cause and cure of back pain remains unknown in the majority of cases.

The massive Quebec study described in chapter 1 found that only short-term bed rest, education about self-care of the back ("back school"), and analgesics have statistically significant efficacy in treatment of acute low back pain. The great majority of therapeutic options that were analyzed in the Quebec study were not found to be effective despite their widespread use.

Myth 11: If your back pain goes on for a long time, you should undergo surgery.

Truth: Surgery is less likely to have a successful outcome in cases of chronic back pain. Often the longer the pain exists, the more difficult it is to determine the cause, since deconditioning and psychological variables continue to complicate the clinical picture. Furthermore most of the indications for spine surgery are fairly clear and are often determined before the situation becomes chronic. Before surgery is considered in a patient with chronic low back pain, the surgeon should consider the role of deconditioning and psychosocial factors. We will address decision-making for surgery in a later chapter.

Myth 12: You must know exactly what is wrong with your back to cure the problem.

Truth: Most back pain actually gets better even if the exact cause is never revealed. In fact there is disagreement among health professionals as to whether some common diagnoses of back pain actually cause pain. Examples of controversial diagnoses include sacroiliac joint dysfunction, facet syndrome, and piriformis syndrome, among others.

Many other diagnosed conditions, which can at times be the source of pain, may actually have nothing to do with the pain in certain individuals. Common examples of this include bulging disc, osteoporosis, degenerative spondylosis, and many others. As an example, in our practice we have seen countless cases in which the back pain had been attributed to a "bulging disc," which was treated surgically only to provide no relief.

Myth 13: Back pain can lead to paralysis if not cured.

Truth: This is false. Again, only in very rare cases will paralysis be a consequence of back pain. Some examples of this might include certain tumors, spinal infection, and unstable spinal fractures. The great majority of back pain is benign and not associated with paralysis, even if left untreated.

Myth 14: If you are athletic and in good shape, you will not have back pain.

Truth: Back pain does not discriminate regarding whom it attacks, and this includes professional athletes. As we write this book, professional hockey player Wayne Gretsky has just returned to full play after being out with a herniated disc. Interestingly he recovered without surgery and returned to play one of his best games. It is true that a well-conditioned athlete with strong abdominal and back muscles may have less chance of sustaining back injury or pain. However, even this is not clear-cut. One study showed that being physically fit did not protect against an occurrence of low back pain. But the physically fit do have a lesser risk of developing chronic back pain, and they will show a more rapid recovery from an acute pain episode.

Other commonly held beliefs about who is at risk for back pain are also questionable. For instance, posture is only a risk factor when it is extremely abnormal. Also there is generally no relationship between height, weight, or body build and low back pain. Leg-length discrepancy has also not been found to predispose a person to low back pain.

Myth 15: A positive, or "abnormal," MRI or CT scan means that you need surgery.

Truth: As stated before, many people with abnormalities found during MRI and CT scans do not have any pain. Therefore "abnormal" findings may not be at all associated with your back pain, nor do they automatically justify surgery.

Myth 16: High-technology scans such as MRI and CT are necessary for your doctor to develop a good treatment approach.

Truth: A good history and physical examination by your doctor should be sufficient to identify the vast majority of patients for whom specific therapy is required. Our Western high-tech medicine approach far too often rushes in with the "million-dollar" evaluation within the early stages of a back-pain problem. Unless there are clear symptom patterns suggesting the need for further radiologic studies, they are usually not necessary. This approach has been well established in the Quebec studies.

Myth 17: If you have back pain and the doctor cannot find the reason, the pain is in your head.

Truth: The pain is never only in your head. Unfortunately there are health professionals who do convey that message to their patients. This can come from the frustration the physician experiences when no diagnosis is found. Doctors are trained to diagnose structural problems and then "fix" them. As we have seen, however, this is the wrong approach to take in a vast majority of cases.

When an individual is complaining of pain, then the pain is certainly real to that individual. The cause may not be apparent to the physician, but this certainly does not mean the pain doesn't exist. It is true that stress, fear, depression, anxiety, and a number of psychosocial factors can contribute to one's perception of pain. The pain, however, is never imaginary. Patients must learn to accept the health profession's inability to identify the exact cause of pain and not obsess by going from doctor to doctor in search of a cause. However, it is important that you see a medical spine specialist if you have persistent symptoms of back pain to rule out any serious problems, such as a tumor or infection.

Myth 18: A heating pad and massage feel good on my back, so it must be helping my back pain.

Truth: Treatments such as heating pads, massage, and ultrasound are generally referred to as passive modality treatments in physical therapy. Although these treatments may feel great (even to someone without back pain!), they are appropriate only on a very limited basis and should always be used as a means of helping to manage the pain while increasing exercise. They are useful in the initial stages of acute back pain and virtually useless in chronic back pain. There is no scientific evidence that these treatments provide any long-term benefit for the pain. Patients commonly tell us that these treatments feel good while they are applied but do not last much beyond the time it takes to drive home.

Myth 19: If you have more back pain when you exercise, then you shouldn't exercise.

Truth: This is another expression of the "let pain be your guide" myth. Beginning on an exercise program after an episode of back pain, or if you suffer from chronic back pain, will almost always result in increased pain at first. This often causes people to stop exercising and return to bed rest. The pain experienced when doing an appropriate exercise program for back pain should be thought of as "good pain." It is the kind of pain that you might experience after going to the gym or doing exercises after you haven't done them for some time. It is a type of soreness and can actually be a signal that you are getting better!

Myth 20: I need to see a specialist to have my back pain evaluated and treated.

Truth: A recent national government study done through the University of Washington Medical School suggests that back pain, in its initial stages, is far too often treated by specialists. Not only is this often not necessary, but it increases costs and can lead to unnecessary treatment, which can be harmful. The early stages of back pain can usually be treated by your family physician in a conservative manner (we will discuss this approach later). Assuming adequate relief has not occurred after about four to six weeks, the talents of a specialist may be useful, whether a physiatrist, orthopedist, or neurosurgeon.

Myth 21: Back problems are about the same all over the world.

Truth: The truth in this area is very revealing! The United States is currently undergoing what many have termed a back-pain epidemic. This epidemic trend appears unique to industrialized countries. In many third-world countries the problem of back pain is virtually nonexistent. In one study of the Arabian culture back problems were not perceived as either an injury or a disabling condition. In addition back problems were not seen as a reason to obtain medical assistance. This is not to say that back pain does not exist in third-world populations. Rather people there with back pain rarely see a need for formal treatment and they do not think that the pain is particularly harmful or a reason to be disabled (e.g., rest). Though there may be a temporary decline in normal activity, people in third-world countries continue to function, probably allowing for a natural rehabilitation of the back pain.

Many researchers believe that these differences can be explained by cultural attitudes toward back pain. This would include how the individual, his or her family, the medical profession, the legal system, and the government view back pain. These cultural differences lead to treating back pain in a different fashion both from a physical and a psychological perspective. Many factors are now being discovered that explain why back pain is such a problem in industrialized countries. These have included such things as fear of the pain, perpetuation of the myths we have discussed, job dissatisfaction, the perception of back pain as an illness, as well as many other nonphysical forces. These will be discussed more fully in later chapters.

Myth 22: Back pain has been a serious concern of the medical profession for a long, long time.

Truth: According to Dr. John Frymoyer, "Prior to 1930 back pain hardly merited attention from the medical profession, except when the cause was traumatic or infectious, or when children had progressive deformities, often due to poliomyelitis." Back pain was considered a normal, nonthreatening part of life. Treatment included slowing down normal activity for a limited time period, then gradually returning to full capabilities.

Now return to the Back Pain IQ Test. Would you change any of your answers now that you've learned some of the truths about back pain?

CHAPTER 4

WHY DO I HURT?

All pain is real. This may seem like an obvious statement, but often people with lingering back pain are treated as if their pain is either imaginary or exaggerated. Pain is a unique problem in medicine because it cannot be directly measured. In other medical problems the doctor usually has objective evidence to evaluate. For example, if you have an infection, your white blood cell count is high. If you have a broken leg, it shows up on an X ray. Back pain is different from these straightforward problems. As we have discussed, in the majority of cases there are no *objective* findings that can explain the pain! Because of this unique situation the back-pain sufferer will often search for the answer to the problem, which can lead to frustration and unnecessary evaluations and treatment.

We often have patients tell us, "My previous doctor told me there is no evidence to explain the pain I am having." The patient feels the pain must be "proven" to the doctor or to family members. We often hear, "If only I had a broken leg with a cast, then they would believe me." The cycle of not being believed and then feeling like you have to prove you are in pain makes you focus on the pain, which increases suffering and leads to *more* pain. The reason doctors may not have believed you is because they ascribed to old, outdated theories of how pain works.

Pain is a subjective experience, and everyone handles it in different ways. Some people are very stoic and reserved about their pain, while other people may react to pain in a more dramatic way. New theories have been developed to explain how and why people experience pain differently. These ideas will be discussed in this chapter.

ACUTE VERSUS CHRONIC PAIN

To understand current theories of pain, it is important to discuss how pain is defined. *Acute pain is currently defined as pain lasting less than approximately three to six months, or pain that is directly related to tissue damage.* This is the kind of pain that you experience when you cut your finger or stick yourself with a needle. *Chronic pain is generally described as pain that lasts more than six months or beyond the point of tissue healing.* This type of pain is often not directly related to identifiable tissue damage. With chronic pain other factors besides tissue damage influence the amount of pain you perceive.

THE SPECIFICITY THEORY OF PAIN

One of the original theories of pain was entitled the specificity theory, proposed by René Descartes in the sixteenth century. This theory proposed that there is a one-to-one relationship between tissue damage or injury and the amount of pain that a person experiences. For instance if you prick your finger with a needle, you would experience a certain amount of pain, whereas if you cut your finger with a knife, you would experience much more pain. *The specificity theory assumes that the intensity of the pain is directly proportional to the amount of injury.*

This theory is generally accurate for acute pain and it does make common sense. The problem is that this theory is still taught in many medical schools as valid for all types of pain, and many physicians still apply the theory in a broad manner. In a large majority of back-pain cases the specificity theory is probably not valid. This theory also presupposes that if surgery or medication can eliminate the *cause* of the pain, then the pain will disappear. As research and clinical practice will support, this is very often not true.

If a doctor applies this theory to your back pain (especially if it is long term or recurrent), then the search for a "problem" to be "fixed" can go on and on. Ultimately if no explanation is found or if the findings don't correlate with how much pain you are expressing, the validity of your pain may be challenged. The real problem is not that you don't have pain but rather that the theory guiding the treatment is outdated.

PROBLEMS WITH THE SPECIFICITY THEORY

This theory has been shown to be inadequate for several reasons. During World War II Dr. Henry Beecher worked with many soldiers who were severely wounded in battle. He discovered that of the wounded men carried into combat hospitals, only one out of three complained of pain enough to require morphine. They either denied having pain or had so little pain that they did not request pain medication. These wounded soldiers were not in a state of shock, nor were they unable to feel pain, since they complained dramatically when their intravenous lines were placed. When Dr. Beecher returned to clinical practice after the war, he noticed that patients with similar wounds from traumas such as a car accident required morphine to alleviate their pain at a much higher rate. In fact in his clinical practice four out of five patients requested morphine for severe pain. Dr. Beecher concluded that this evidence shows there is no simple, direct relationship between a wound and the pain experienced. In his observations the injury to the wounded soldier had a different "meaning" to the soldier than it did to the civilian. To the soldier it meant "release, thankfulness at his escape alive from the battle field, even euphoria." Alternatively the injury to the civilian and the subsequent major surgery was "a depressing, calamitous event" (Beecher 1959, page 165). The differences in the situations actually caused people with similar wounds to experience different levels of pain. This was a case where the specificity theory did not even hold up for an acute pain situation.

Another finding that discounted the specificity theory was that of phantom-limb pain. Many times patients who undergo amputation of a limb report still experiencing sensations from the limb that has been amputated. They report feeling the limb move through space in much the same way as the normal limb used to feel. In some cases of amputation there will occur a painful phantom-limb syndrome in which the patient feels severe pain in the amputated limb even though the limb no longer exists. Of course the specificity theory cannot account for these findings because there is no ongoing tissue damage evoking the pain.

One other finding that the specificity theory cannot explain is that of hypnosis used for anesthesia or pain relief. It has been found that people under hypnosis can sustain high levels of pain under which they would normally cry out or withdraw. Major surgery on every part of the body has been carried out on patients in which the only anesthesia was hypnosis. Although the mechanisms for hypnosis are unclear, the evidence demonstrates that tissue damage or injury does not always relate to the amount of pain experienced.

THE GATE-CONTROL THEORY OF PAIN

Because of the above-mentioned findings, a new theory of pain was developed that could explain these results. In the early 1960s Drs. Ronald Melzack and Patrick Wall developed the "gate control" theory of pain. This theory is very complex and attempts to explain on a physiological level the findings discussed above.

The gate-control theory suggests that pain can be thought of as being divided into two components, which are processed separately. These are the peripheral-nervous-system component (outside the brain and spinal cord) and the central-nervous-system component (within the brain). Nerve endings have pain receptors, which detect painful stimuli and transmit them through nerve fibers to the spinal cord. The peripheral nerves, which are sensory nerves, also carry a variety of other common sensations including temperature, light touch, and vibration, as well as other sensory phenomenon. The nerve endings that detect pain are present in many structures found in the back, including the discs, the vertebral bodies, the facet joints, and multiple muscular and ligamentous structures that make up the spine. When one of these structures is irritated, inflamed, or mechanically malfunctioning, the sensation of pain will typically be transmitted by the pain fibers of the peripheral nerves to the spinal cord and on to the brain.

The gate-control theory also proposes that there are "gates" on the bundles of nerve fibers in the spinal cord between the peripheral nervous system and the brain. These "spinal nerve gates" can either open to allow pain impulses to freely move from the peripheral nerves to the brain, or they can close to stop the pain signals from reaching the brain. The opening and closing of the pain gates is influenced by several things, which will be discussed later.

When the sensation reaches the brain, it undergoes another type of processing while in the central nervous system. Thus the pain sensation actually goes through two distinct types of processing, and the experience of the pain is a combination of these two factors. The first, in the peripheral component, is generally relative to the amount of tissue damage (as in acute pain). The second is the central component, and this can greatly affect the pain experience.

The opening and closing of the nerve gates really determines how much of the pain impulse is experienced. This is dependent upon several things. The theory proposes that the brain can send signals down to the spinal nerve gates, which actually close, causing a decrease in pain perception. Thus, when the gates are fully open, you will experience the pain at its highest degree, and when the gates are fully closed, you will experience pain at its lowest degree. The pain gates can be thought of as the "volume control knob" on your pain, which is controlled by the brain. The pain input from the peripheral nerves can be shut off or on, or turned up or down by the pain-gates system.

OPENING AND CLOSING THE PAIN GATES

Factors that open and close the pain gates can be divided into sensory (or physical), emotional, and cognitive (thought) areas. Sensory factors that open the pain gates include injury, inactivity, long-term narcotic use, poor body mechanics, and poor pacing of your activities. Emotional factors that open the pain gates include depression, anger, anxiety, stress, frustration, hopelessness, and helplessness. Thoughts that can open the pain gates include focusing on the pain, having no outside interests, worrying about the pain, and thinking that your future is a catastrophe.

Alternatively there are several factors in each of these areas that can help close the gates and thus decrease your pain and suffering. Sensory factors that help close the gates can include increasing your activity, short-term use of pain medication, aerobic exercise, and relaxation training. Emotional factors that close the pain gates include decreasing depression, having a positive attitude, being reassured that the pain is not harmful, stress management, and feeling like you are in control of your pain and your life. Thoughts that can close the pain gates include distraction from the pain, outside interests, and other thoughts that help you cope. Figure 4-1 depicts how these spinal nerve gates open and close affecting the experience of pain in the brain. In the examples of Dr. Beecher discussed above, the meaning of the situation in which the pain was experienced was the key element in whether the nerve gates were open or closed. The meaning of the injury to the combat soldiers was more positive in that they were escaping with their lives; hence the pain gates were closed. Similar injuries to civilians held a negative meaning, which opened the pain gates.

The following two examples help illustrate how pain is influenced by thoughts, feelings, and the situation in which it occurs. The first example illustrates closing the pain gates and decreasing pain, while the second example illustrates opening the pain gates and increasing pain.

If a tight clothespin is placed on your arm and you are in-

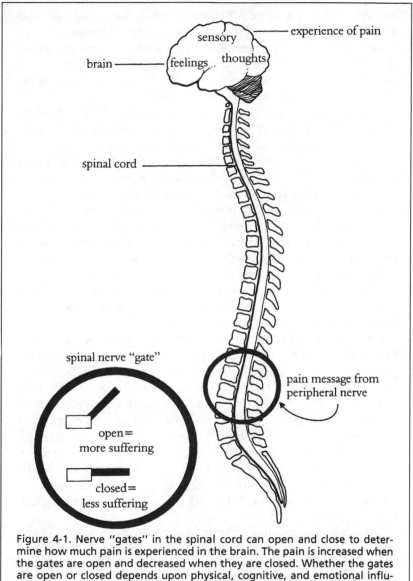

Figure 4-1. Nerve "gates" in the spinal cord can open and close to determine how much pain is experienced in the brain. The pain is increased when the gates are open and decreased when they are closed. Whether the gates are open or closed depends upon physical, cognitive, and emotional influences. Illustration provided courtesy of Century City Hospital, Los Angeles.

structed to leave it there for the entire day, the initial pain you experience would be quite severe as the clothespin compresses your skin and muscles. Peripheral nerve fibers sense this pressure and transmit a pain message to the spinal cord and then to the brain. The pain is initially perceived as fairly proportional to the pressure on the skin.

After a short while the message of pain, which continues to come to the brain, will be decreased by a closing of the pain gates. The reason is as follows: The brain begins to view the pain message as nonharmful, as you would expect a clothespin on your arm to be. The pressure is painful, but it is not harming you in any way (it is not causing tissue damage). Subsequently the pain message is given less attention by the brain and thereby brought to consciousness at a much less intense level. In brief summary, since the brain knows that the clothespin, which has to stay on the arm all day long, is of no great significance and has no potential to cause damage to the body, it turns down the volume on the pain and you experience it as much less intense. In fact after about thirty minutes you would barely perceive any pain at all.

Does this mean that you no longer have pain? Actually the clothespin is still compressing the skin and muscles, and the peripheral nerves are still sending pain messages to the spinal cord. But the brain is processing the signals much differently now. Now the signal is felt as a mild discomfort rather than "pain," resulting in a much decreased level of suffering.

The second example was a clinical experience of Dr. Sinel at Cornell University Medical Center. A woman complained of headaches, which were described as severely painful and debilitating, preventing her from getting through the day without taking narcotic pain medicine. The headaches had occurred over the previous month.

A thorough neurologic examination and history was entirely normal. After speaking with the patient for some time it became more clear why the headaches were occurring. When questioned about the stress in her life, the patient reported that her husband had recently been diagnosed with an inoperable brain tumor. She said his initial symptoms were headaches, for which he had failed to seek medical advice for three months. A brain tumor was ultimately diagnosed after an MRI was obtained, and the patient's husband died shortly thereafter.

It became apparent that this woman had an extreme fear that she, too, had a brain tumor and that this was causing the headaches. This belief was creating intense suffering, which in turn made the headaches worse. An MRI was obtained and shown to be negative, and the diagnosis of tension headaches was further confirmed. The patient was extensively reassured as to the benign nature of her headaches. After experiencing tremendous relief that the headaches were not the result of something harmful, the patient's symptoms began to dissipate rapidly. Within two days she was managing the headache pain with no more than nonprescription medicine. After receiving some stress-management training over the next few weeks the patient was entirely off pain medicine and the headaches had remitted.

As can be seen by the two examples above, how your brain assesses the pain situation is critical in the experience of suffering. In the first example, we saw that the pain message from the clothespin was interpreted by the brain as nonthreatening and subsequently decreased. In the second example the pain message from the tension headache was interpreted by the patient as dangerous and life-threatening. This resulted in an amplification of the pain and suffering. This pain and suffering diminished after the patient's beliefs about the pain were changed through reassurance.

We see examples of this on a daily basis in clinical practice. Patients who have seen doctor after doctor and have been given diagnosis after diagnosis are reassured that their back pain is benign and in many cases a normal part of life. This does not mean there is no pain. Rather it means that the pain is not signaling harm to the back. It is like having a tension headache in your back. If the patient accepts the reassurance and changes his or her beliefs about the pain, tremendous relief is often experienced.

What is the relevance of the gate-control theory to back pain? Based on our clinical experience and the research literature, we strongly believe that back pain is very often amplified in the brain, causing greater pain perception and more suffering than is necessary. Amplification of the pain is often a consequence of the patient's perceived meaning of his or her back pain. This is commonly associated with fear of an underlying disease, anticipated surgery, disability, financial stress, fear of movement or injury, as well as other factors. All of these things enhance the negative meaning of the pain, making you experience more pain than you should.

As we have discussed in the chapter on medical myths, in the vast majority of cases there is no serious underlying pathology in back pain. We very often see that after reassurance that the pain is benign and the encouragement that "hurt does not equal harm" there is a tremendous relief in patients. This is the effect of attitudinal healing in pain management whereby the ability of the brain to decrease the pain is greatly enhanced.

CHRONIC PAIN

The gate-control theory also helps explain why chronic pain can often be very stressful and associated with negative emotions, including depression and anxiety. The pain receptors and nerve fibers that transmit more acute pain generally go directly from the receptor area (for example your back) to the spinal cord and on to the thalamus and cortex in your brain.

The pain system that is responsible for the perception of chronic pain can take a different route. These are the slow nerve fibers, which transmit pain often described as dull, aching, burning, and cramping. These fibers go from the receptor site to the hypothalamus (which is the brain structure that controls stress hormones) and then through the limbic system (which is the brain structure that controls emotions). It is theorized that the different nerve route that slow (chronic) pain takes helps explain why stress and depression/anxiety are often part of a chronic pain problem. You may have experienced some of these other factors of pain if you suffer from constant, chronic back pain. These issues will be discussed more fully in the last section.

PART II

EVALUATION OF
YOUR BACK PAIN

CHAPTER 5

GETTING TO KNOW YOUR SPINE

This chapter is being provided as a brief and simple overview of the structure of the spine. Most people have no idea what their spine looks like, how it is meant to function, or the component parts that make up their back. This chapter will acquaint you with your spine. It will help you to understand the various terms that your doctor might use in discussing your back problem. Health care professionals often forget to use language that is interpretable by anyone but themselves. This chapter will help you to "speak their language," which will increase your understanding and help decrease miscommunication. Overall this will help you obtain better, more cost-effective treatment for your back-pain problem.

In learning about your spine it is important not to succumb to the "medical-student syndrome," in which a little knowledge actually makes things worse. We have had patients learn about their spine structure only to begin to worry that every part we had discussed with them was "weakened," or malfunctioning. Throughout this chapter it should be kept in mind that:

In the vast majority of back-pain cases no structural problem will be identified.

PURPOSE

The spine is designed to support your upper body, protect your spinal cord, provide flexibility, and serve as an attachment point for muscles and ligaments. It provides strength and stability for the upper body and has powerful shock-absorbing capabilities. It is without question one of the most magnificent structures in nature.

STRUCTURE

The Spinal Column

As can be seen in figure 5-1, the back is generally divided into three curves, called the cervical curve (your neck), the thoracic curve (your midback), and the lumbar curve (your lower back). As seen from the side, the back is actually S-shaped as a result of these three natural curves. The spine is made up of vertebrae, which are the bones of the spine. There are a total of twenty-four vertebrae in your back. There are seven vertebrae in the cervical part of the spine making up your neck. The cervical vertebrae support the weight of your head and protect the nerves that come from your brain to the rest of your body. In medical jargon the cervical vertebrae are generally referred to as C1 to C7, with C1 being the first cervical vertebrae just under your head.

The middle part of the back is composed of twelve thoracic vertebrae. These are referred to as T1 to T12. Lastly there are the five vertebrae in the lower back, referred to as the lumbar spine. As you might have guessed, these are referred to as L1 to L5.

The Vertebrae

As mentioned above, the vertebrae are actually the bones of the back. Each vertebra has basically three parts: the vertebral body, the transverse process, and the spinous process. Figure 5-2 depicts a single vertebra from a side view, whereas figure 5-3 is a view from above. The vertebral body is the large part that surrounds and protects the spinal canal. The spinous process is the part of the vertebrae that can be felt as the "bony bumps" protruding from your back. Lastly the transverse process provides an area for attachment of the muscles that con-

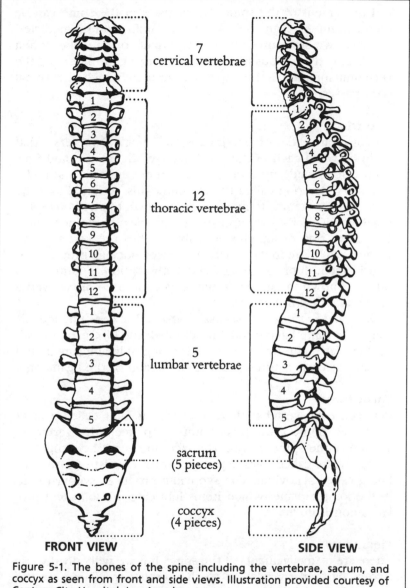

7
cervical vertebrae

12
thoracic vertebrae

5
lumbar vertebrae

sacrum
(5 pieces)

coccyx
(4 pieces)

FRONT VIEW

SIDE VIEW

Figure 5-1. The bones of the spine including the vertebrae, sacrum, and coccyx as seen from front and side views. Illustration provided courtesy of Century City Hospital, Los Angeles.

trol movement of the spine. Other parts of the spine can be seen in figures 5-2 and 5-3. Notice the lamina and the pedicles, as these two structures will be important to remember when we discuss the various types of back surgery. In figure 5-3 the vertebral foramen is the opening through which the spinal cord passes.

The Discs

The discs are the cushioning pads, or "shock absorbers," that lie in between each of the vertebrae (see figures 5-4 and 5-5). Each disc is made up of a spongy center (the nucleus) and a tougher outer ring called the annulus. This design allows the hard, bony vertebrae to move back and forth to give your spine flexibility. The discs are approximately one-quarter-inch thick. The outer ring or annulus actually attaches the vertebrae together, while the inner spongy center or nucleus provides for nourishment, lubrication, and shock absorption. A "functional unit" is shown in figure 5-4, which is composed of two vertebrae and a disc in between.

One can see from this discussion that a disc does not actually "slip," as some have termed it, although the disc can "bulge" or "herniate" through the posterior longitudinal ligament and irritate nerve structures (see the discussion of the ligaments).

Facet Joints

Between each vertebra there is a gliding joint called a facet joint (see figure 5-4). Facet joints help keep the vertebrae aligned as the spine moves. The facet joints are held together by ligaments called joint capsules, which consist of a smooth lining called synovium. The synovium produces synovial fluid in the joint capsule, which helps lubricate the joint and provides nourishment.

Ligaments

There are many ligaments of the spine, but we will only discuss two as particularly relevant to this discussion. These are the anterior (toward the front) longitudinal ligament and the posterior (toward the rear) longitudinal ligament (see figure 5-6).

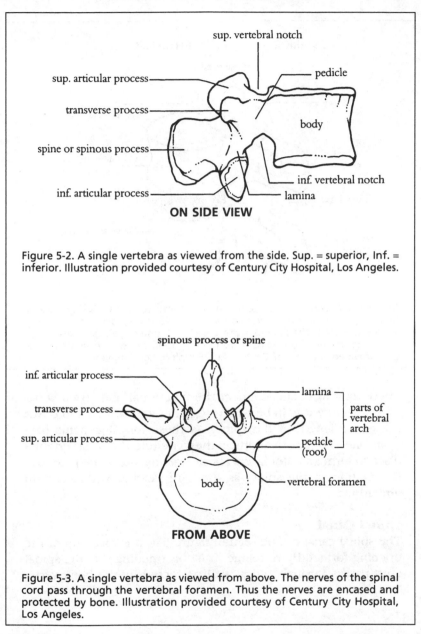

ON SIDE VIEW

Figure 5-2. A single vertebra as viewed from the side. Sup. = superior, Inf. = inferior. Illustration provided courtesy of Century City Hospital, Los Angeles.

FROM ABOVE

Figure 5-3. A single vertebra as viewed from above. The nerves of the spinal cord pass through the vertebral foramen. Thus the nerves are encased and protected by bone. Illustration provided courtesy of Century City Hospital, Los Angeles.

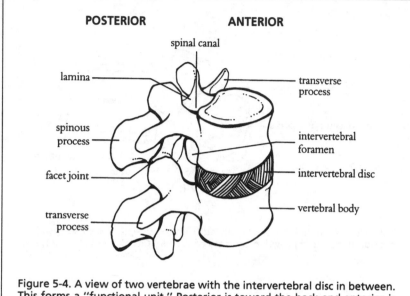

POSTERIOR   **ANTERIOR**

spinal canal

lamina

transverse process

spinous process

intervertebral foramen

facet joint

intervertebral disc

transverse process

vertebral body

Figure 5-4. A view of two vertebrae with the intervertebral disc in between. This forms a "functional unit." Posterior is toward the back and anterior is toward the front. The spinous process are the "bumps" you can feel on your back. The nerves of the spinal cord pass through the spinal canal. Illustration provided courtesy of Century City Hospital, Los Angeles.

These long ligaments connect the functional units (two vertebrae with one disc in between) together and run up and down the entire length of the spine. As these long ligaments pass from one vertebra to another, they encircle the intervertebral discs to form an outer layer. These large ligaments help control the motion of the spine, as they are flexible within certain limitations.

Spinal Canal

The spinal canal can be seen in figure 5-4. It is made up of the opening formed by vertebrae. It is this opening that the spinal cord passes through and is well protected by the bony vertebrae.

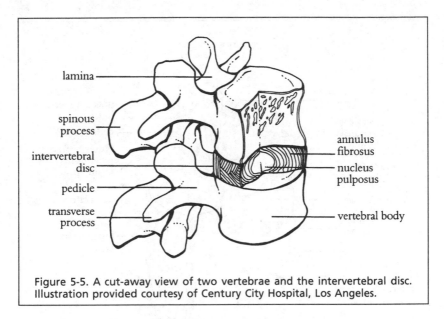

Figure 5-5. A cut-away view of two vertebrae and the intervertebral disc. Illustration provided courtesy of Century City Hospital, Los Angeles.

The Sacrum and Coccyx

After the five lumbar vertebrae there are five more vertebrae that are fused (attached) together. These five vertebrae, which can be seen in figure 5-7, make up the sacrum, and this forms the back part of the pelvis. In the vast majority of people there are five lumbar vertebrae and, then, the five fused sacral vertebrae. In some people the sixth lumbar vertebra does not fuse with the sacrum. This results in six lumbar vertebrae and only four fused sacral vertebrae. However, this condition is rarely the cause of any back problems.

The last structure of the "bony" part of the spine is the coccyx. This consists of three to five small vertebrae that are attached to the bottom of the sacrum.

Sacroiliac Joints

The sacroiliac joints are the joints that attach the sacrum (*sacro-*) to the iliac bones of the pelvis. This can also be seen in figure 5-7. The iliac bones of the pelvis are those that can be felt as your hips. Many years ago it was thought that problems

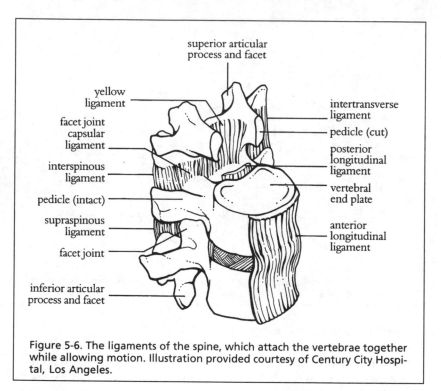

Figure 5-6. The ligaments of the spine, which attach the vertebrae together while allowing motion. Illustration provided courtesy of Century City Hospital, Los Angeles.

with the sacroiliac joint (e.g., misalignment) were the source of many cases of back pain. This is no longer thought to be the case.

Nerves

The spinal cord is made up of nerves, which extend from the brain into the spinal canal and then out to various parts of the body. The spinal canal is formed by the large part of the vertebrae as well as other structures. It is essentially a tube that is partly filled with a fluid substance (cerebrospinal fluid). The spinal cord (the bundles of nerves) is protected within this fluid. As mentioned above, one of the primary purposes of the spine is to protect the nerves in the spinal cord.

In simple terms we see two common "nerve pain" problems

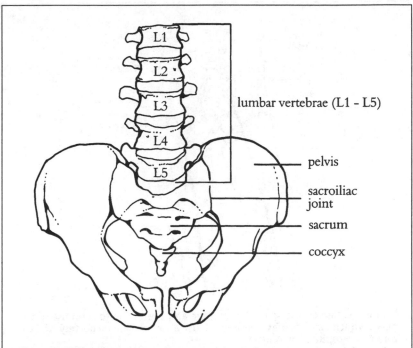

Figure 5-7. The lumbar vertebrae, sacrum, and coccyx as viewed from the front. Illustration provided courtesy of Century City Hospital, Los Angeles.

in the spine, one much more common than the other. These are herniated or bulging disc(s) either in the cervical spine or the lumbar spine. Disc herniation in the cervical spine is less common and can cause pain down one or both arms (radiculopathy) because the nerves that supply the arms and hands are being "pinched" or compressed by the disc problem in the neck.

The second problem occurs with a disc(s) in the lumbar spine and is by far the most common spine problem. A disc bulge or herniation can press upon one or more nerves, causing pain to radiate down one or both legs. This radiating pain is referred to as sciatica due to the involvement of the sciatic nerve.

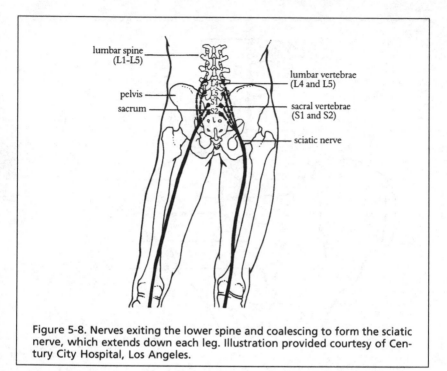

Figure 5-8. Nerves exiting the lower spine and coalescing to form the sciatic nerve, which extends down each leg. Illustration provided courtesy of Century City Hospital, Los Angeles.

Muscles

There are many muscles involved in the function of the spine. These include muscles in the back as well as in the abdominal area. Only the most important muscles will be discussed here.

The erector spinae muscles are those that run down the back on either side of the spine. They are the ones that patients commonly say are "tense" or "in spasm" as part of their back-pain complaint. Just under these long muscles are medium-length muscles that stretch from one vertebra to the next. Under these muscles are even shorter muscles, which attach to the facet joints. All of these muscles are at the rear of the spine. There is another muscle (the psoas muscle), which runs from the front and side of the lower back, across the hip joint, and attaches to the very upper part of the thighbone (femur).

In addition the muscles of the abdomen are important to the forward movement of the spine, as there are actually very few muscles that attach to the front of the vertebrae. The abdominal muscles provide important support to the spine.

CHAPTER 6

DIAGNOSIS IN BACK PAIN

It is important for you to understand the common diagnoses in back pain in order to prevent the unnecessary fear these labels often provoke. Before proceeding with this discussion, we will outline the general purpose of diagnosis in medicine, how this purpose can cause problems when applied to back pain, and reasons for incorrect diagnoses when dealing with back pain.

THE PURPOSE OF DIAGNOSIS IN MEDICINE

In traditional medicine the three principles of treatment are "diagnosis, diagnosis, and diagnosis." This is because it is generally held in medicine that if you don't know what is wrong, you cannot give proper treatment. The problem with back pain is that one cannot always come up with an exact anatomical diagnosis. In fact, as discussed earlier, an exact diagnosis for acute back pain is possible in only about 10 to 15 percent of cases. In chronic back-pain cases the percentage may be even lower! Therefore in most cases a physician's job is to rule out certain diagnoses that can be serious life-threatening illnesses that need immediate attention, such as tumors, infections, progressive nerve-root damage, or significant spinal instability that might put the spinal cord in danger. You can be assured that modern clinical examination and diagnostic techniques are very good at determining these rare conditions. In addition these techniques are also excellent at determining back-pain conditions due to such things as a disc herniation or spinal stenosis. Even so, as we shall see in this chapter and the next, these diagnostic techniques must be used very carefully, as they can easily lead to incorrect treatment. Once a serious condition is ruled out, your doctor will often be left with back pain of essentially unknown origin in precise terms. Still, it is important to remember:

> **You can be reassured that treatment for back pain can be very effective even without knowing the exact cause.**

As we have discussed in previous chapters, this is what makes back pain unique in medicine. Although we can't always make a very specific diagnosis, we can go ahead and treat someone successfully.

You should be aware that people will often feel the need to have some kind of diagnosis even if there is little evidence that the diagnosis is causing their pain (or even whether such a condition actually exists). This "need for a diagnosis" affects both medical and other health care approaches. This may explain in part why people are drawn to alternative health care practitioners, as these groups are usually able to come up with a specific diagnosis, whether it is correct or not. People are told that a joint is out of place in the spine or some other explanation for their back pain. The patient will then feel reassured that "this person knows exactly what is wrong with my back and can fix it."

One problem with a patient's need for a diagnosis is that doctors will often attempt to comply by focusing on some anatomical variant noticed on a very sophisticated imaging study. This finding may be nothing more than the normal aging change in the spine and often will have absolutely nothing to do with the back pain. This can lead to fear, suffering, and unnecessary treatment. It is amazing to see the impact on people when they are told they have a "slipped disc"; suddenly they see themselves as a "cripple," somehow damaged and different from the way they were before they found out about the slipped disc. As we shall see, research is showing us that much of what were previously thought to be "significant" findings on these tests are actually "nonsignificant" parts of the normal aging process.

THE REASONS FOR INCORRECT DIAGNOSIS IN BACK PAIN

We feel that there are three common reasons that people are given incorrect diagnoses. First a structural diagnosis for the back pain is made based on an imaging scan. This is part of a patient's need for a diagnosis and the doctor's need to give one. The doctor feels that showing the patient something like degenerative changes on an X ray will serve the purpose of explaining the pain even if the findings have absolutely nothing to do with the pain. What the doctor does not take into account is the devastating impact such findings can have on a person, who now thinks his or her spine is "damaged." For instance imagine how upsetting it would be for a forty-five-year-old man with low back pain to see arthritic changes on an X ray. Research shows that such changes are commonly seen in a large percentage of patients without back pain and in most cases have no significance at all. Even so, the physician or other practitioner, in an attempt to give the patient a diagnosis, will point out the degenerative arthritic change and say that it is the cause of the pain.

In many patients this can create extensive problems. First they see a structural problem that they believe is causing the pain, a problem for which there is "no cure." Second, by a diagnosis of this as "degenerative," they believe the problem will get worse over time.

A second common reason that physicians give incorrect anatomical diagnoses to patients is ignorance on the part of the practitioner. It has only been in the recent decade that we have begun to appreciate the extent of asymptomatic findings (findings that do not cause symptoms) on sophisticated imaging studies, such as on MRI. More and more research is showing the high prevalence of disc herniations, minor scoliosis, and other radiographic abnormalities that don't necessarily have any correlation to a patient's clinical symptoms. These findings are now being understood as normal variants and not anything significant.

A third common reason is that most physicians and practitioners who diagnose and treat back pain do not have a sufficient appreciation for the impact of psychological, emotional, and social factors in back pain. These issues are discussed extensively later in this chapter as well as in other chapters. An example of such a condition is "stress-related back pain," in which the primary factor in the pain is thought to be emotional. Another example is chronic back pain that has gone on for more than about six months. If the practitioner is not aware of these influences on back pain, the likelihood of an incorrect diagnosis along with inappropriate treatment is very great. Of course there will be no adequate response to this incorrect "structural approach" if these other factors are primary.

With these issues in mind we will review some of the most common diagnoses in back pain, including those from both traditional medicine and other, nontraditional areas.

DIAGNOSES IN BACK PAIN

Cauda Equina Syndrome
Cauda equina syndrome is a very rare occurrence in which there is a compression of the fluid-filled sac of the lower portion of the spine that contains the nerve roots after the spinal cord ends and the nerves continue. Some of the nerves that continue at the lower part of the spine supply the function to the bowel and bladder as well as the sensation to the entire area around the groin and anal region. When these nerve roots are compressed, the individual might experience loss of function of the bowel or bladder. This might include the inability to control or initiate urination as well as loss of feeling during a bowel movement or loss of ability to initiate or control a bowel

movement. Furthermore there may be loss of male erectile function and loss of sensation to the entire groin area.

If a patient notices any of the symptoms of cauda equina syndrome, this does constitute a medical emergency that needs immediate attention. The treatment of cauda equina syndrome involves surgically removing whatever might be compressing the sacral nerve roots. It is critical that the treatment of this syndrome take place immediately upon diagnosis, because the loss of neurologic function to the bowel and bladder can be permanent if not corrected within less than twenty-four to forty-eight hours.

Herniated Disc/Sciatica

As discussed previously, the discs lie between the vertebrae and act as cushions for the spine. A disc bulge or herniation occurs when the soft gel-like material of the nucleus pulposus pushes out from between the vertebrae. When a disc bulges toward the back of your body (posterior) and breaks through the annulus fibrosis, it is referred to as a herniation, although frequently the nucleus of the disc just bulges out and does not actually break through the outer ring (annulus fibrosus) or ligament. This is referred to as a "bulging" disc and is seen very commonly on MRI scans.

The bulging disc does not usually cause any symptoms, as there is no irritation or compression of nerve roots of the spine. In fact after the age of forty the incidence of bulging discs is seen in 50 percent or more of all MRI scans in individuals without symptoms.

In a herniated disc the gel-like material of the nucleus pulposus can press against a nearby spinal nerve and cause the pain typically referred to as sciatica. "Sciatic" pain occurs when the nerves of the lumbar spine are "compressed" (pushed against) by a herniated disc where the nerves exit through the vertebral canal. The nerves supply the sensation and strength to the leg as well as the reflexes of the leg, extending all the way down to the foot.

More than 90 percent of all herniated discs in the lumbar spine occur at the levels of L4–5 and L5–S1, with the former being more prevalent. Typically sciatic pain occurs in the buttocks, back of the thigh and calf, and occasionally going down to the foot and heel. The nerve root is most commonly "compressed" but not "compromised" (in other words, it is irritated but still works). Occasionally, however, there is enough compression of the nerve to result in decreases in strength, sensation, and reflex. This condition may require surgical intervention, although the great majority of disc herniations do respond to nonsurgical, conservative management.

Since the advent of MRI examination we are finding a very high incidence of herniated discs in patients without back or sciatic pain. It has been shown that over 35 percent of individuals without symptoms over the age of forty are found to have herniated discs by MRI finding. We frequently see patients who have been given a diagnosis of a herniated disc when in fact it has nothing to do with their pain and does not correlate whatsoever with the clinical history and examination findings. In these cases it is unfortunate that the patient has been alarmed by the diagnosis when it actually is not playing a role in the pain. Even worse is when a patient undergoes unnecessary surgery for a herniated disc and his or her symptoms continue unchanged after the operation. It is extremely important that the evaluating physician be aware of the frequency of disc herniations that do not cause symptoms and have a high level of skill in correlating MRI findings with the physical examination and history.

The physical examination is a standard part of the evaluation in a patient with back and/or sciatic-type pain. It is important for patients to be aware of this in order to avoid a doctor giving a diagnosis by merely looking at an MRI scan without a proper history and examination. The highlights of the physical examination include the following:

1. A straight-leg-raise test is performed with a patient lying flat on his or her back with feet extended fully on the examination table. The examiner then lifts one leg at a time and assesses the onset of pain down the leg (sciatica) as the leg is raised. In a typical disc herniation pain

will shoot down the affected leg when it is raised between 30 and 70 degrees. The reason for this is that the nerve roots at the spinal cord level are stretched and put under increased tension.

2. We also occasionally see pain radiating down the involved leg when the opposite leg is raised, often indicating the presence of a disc fragment. A disc fragment is seen when a piece of the herniated disc breaks off and floats into the vertebral canal, compressing the nerve root.

3. The straight-leg-raise test is usually complemented by a test known as Lasegue's, which involves bringing the patient's ankle and foot up toward the knee, thereby putting further stress on the nerve roots of the spine. A simple way to understand this test is to imagine the sciatic nerve as being like a string extending from the spinal cord in the back to the entire lower extremity to the tip of the toes. When this nerve is put under tension by extending the straight leg upward and further pulling back on the ankle (like stretching the string), it causes irritation at the nerve root and reproduction of the pain.

4. A detailed neurologic examination of the lower extremities (hip, thigh, leg, and foot) is required to assess the degree of nerve compromise that might be caused by a herniated disc. This consists of testing the sensation throughout the leg and foot, often performed by moving both a cotton swab and a pinwheel over the surface of the skin.

   The reflexes at the knee and back of the ankle both correspond to specific nerve levels of the spine and are typically evaluated in a patient with sciatica or disc herniation.

5. Finally, and most importantly, is testing the motor strength of all the individual muscle groups of the lower extremity, again each of which corresponds to a specific nerve-root level in the spine.

This kind of physical examination will help determine the "level" of the disc problem, which refers to the area of spine where the disc injury or herniation has occurred. Your doctor can fairly accurately detect what level of the spine has been injured by looking for the different patterns of symptoms and examination findings in your lower extremities.

Typically the pain of herniated discs is increased upon bending and sitting, as this tends to significantly increase the pressure in the discs, although this is not always seen clinically. The physical examination should also include range of motion of the lumbar spine as well as manual examination for evidence of spasm or tenderness along the course of the nerve root going down the leg.

Several diagnostic tests help in evaluating the presence of a herniated disc. Currently MRI evaluation allows an excellent visualization of the disc and nerve-root structures, although CT scan and myelogram are certainly commonly used and can often adequately assess the presence of a disc herniation. Electrodiagnostic studies (to be discussed further in the testing chapter) are utilized to test for the presence of nerve (root) irritation. Testing always needs to be correlated well with the patient's history and clinical examination.

The diagnosis of disc herniation is fairly common when patients have sciatic pain. However, the presence of sciatica without loss of motor strength, sensation, or reflexes frequently does not require further diagnostic evaluation and can be diagnosed purely on the basis of history and physical examination. There has been a tremendous overutilization of MRI and other diagnostic tests in evaluating these conditions. This diagnosis should not require extensive diagnostic testing unless surgery is being considered as part of the treatment, and this should occur very infrequently. The great majority of patients with disc herniations have been shown to recover with conservative management.

A herniated disc, even in the presence of nerve-root compression, is very rarely a serious problem. It should be considered serious if the compression of the nerve roots leads to a progressive weakening of the muscles or loss of sensation in the lower extremity, or causes a cauda equina syndrome. However, in most cases the herniated disc merely causes some pain and occasionally some very mild neurologic deficit, such as a mild sensory loss, reflex loss, or minimal weakness, which frequently return as the patient recovers. The natural history of disc herniation is quite favorable, with the great majority of patients showing spontaneous recovery within two to three months with conservative management.

A typical course of evaluation and treatment of a disc herniation is as follows. A thorough physical examination and history should be done by the doctor in which it is also determined whether the symptoms are worsening or beginning to get better. This is one of the most important questions in evaluating disc herniation and/or sciatica because there is never a need for further diagnostic testing when someone is improving.

The time course of symptoms is relevant because when a patient presents with symptoms of recent onset (less than one month), it is reasonable for the physician to observe the patient and begin conservative management, as the natural history will likely lead to improvement. We very rarely order MRI or other radiographic tests unless a surgical option is being considered. The only considerations for this in the first month of symptoms might be progressive nerve compression with increasing weakness of the leg or severely progressive intolerable pain, unresponsive to medication. We will employ conservative therapy consisting of physical therapy, exercises (which will be described later), and anti-inflammatory medication to reduce the swelling of the nerve root.

In the case of more chronic symptoms or chronically recurring symptoms, the patient should be advised that the likelihood of progression of these symptoms is minimal. In these cases it is perfectly acceptable for an individual either to attempt continued conservative management or simply to live with the symptoms if the level is acceptable. This level of symptoms might be controlled with occasional use of medication, such as an over-the-counter anti-inflammatory, and occasional limitations of certain activities (e.g., aggressive sporting activities, heavy lifting and twisting). However, even if the indi-

vidual desires to pursue these activities, which might potentially aggravate the underlying disc herniation, he or she is
usually not in any danger of doing any harm other than experiencing persistent pain.

We have had many patients in our practice who have returned to such things as heavy weight lifting, contact sports,
and almost any occupation following disc herniation, without
ever undergoing surgical intervention. Many of these patients
have seen improvement of their symptoms over time and others simply go on tolerating the ongoing pain and discomfort
with occasional minimal weakness or loss of sensation.

Pinched Nerve, Nerve Compression, Spinal Cord Compression

Pinched nerve is a commonly used term to represent what we
would call a sciatica or irritation of a branch of the sciatic
nerve, as was discussed above. The irritation could be caused
by a piece of the soft portion of the disc being too close to the
nerve, or it can actually be caused by mechanical compression,
or both.

Spinal cord compression is something that very rarely occurs
since the spinal cord, as such, ends 4 to 5 inches above where
95 percent of disc ruptures or disc herniations occur. Spinal
cord compression is seen in the very rare disc herniations that
occur in the thoracic spine. The reason disc herniations are so
rare in the thoracic spine is the increased stability in this area
due to the rib attachments.

Sprain-Strain

In clinical practice the "sprain-strain" injury is probably the
most common cause of back pain. Although the terms are
often used together (a "sprain-strain injury"), we will differentiate the two in terms of presumed etiology. This is somewhat
of an academic point, as the symptoms and treatment are essentially the same.

In the most straightforward terms, a *sprain* is an injury to a
muscle, ligament, or tendon (which attaches a muscle to
bone). This usually occurs as a result of a fairly identifiable

acute injury, such as a car or sports accident. For example a muscle might be stretched beyond its natural limit, causing some bleeding and inflammation. In response to this injury the muscle will tighten up. Symptoms might include pain of immediate onset or pain gradually worsening over hours or days following the injury. Often there will be muscle spasms in the back as the result either of an injured muscle or of the muscles tightening in response to other structures having been injured, such as ligaments or tendons. Movement will usually make the pain more severe. One common pattern is to notice the pain being worse in the morning and then improving with some activity over the course of the day. The muscles seem to warm up and the discomfort subsides.

A *strain*, in our opinion, is an injury similar to a sprain except that it occurs over a period of time as a result of a confluence of different factors. These might include such things as very poor posture, lifting incorrectly over and over again, physical deconditioning, and incorrect repetitive motion of the back. In a strain injury any one event would not be enough to cause an injury to the muscle or other structures. It is a buildup of these types of maneuvers or events that can cause the injury. This can lead to a type of chronic situation in which a ligament or muscle remains inflamed at a certain level over a period of time. Clinical manifestations are similar to that of a sprain except for the clear-cut, identifiable precipitant.

It should be noted that other professionals define these terms somewhat differently. Many will define a sprain as an injury to a ligament or tendon and a strain as an injury to a muscle. As can be seen from the above, our definitions are slightly different. These slightly different definitions have no impact on how the condition is evaluated and treated.

Most practitioners will use the term *sprain-strain* because determining the factors that caused the injury are not clear or because there are both types of injury occurring simultaneously. An example of this might be the "weekend warrior" athlete who sits at a desk all week only to go out for an aggressive game of basketball on Saturday. The weekend injury during the game (sprain) is superimposed on the poor posture and deconditioning occurring during the week (strain). As the diagnosis and treatment issues are essentially the same, we will use the term *sprain-strain* from here on.

The diagnosis is usually based upon the absence of other findings that suggest any type of nerve-root irritation. The diagnosis is also based upon the history of an event, or repeated events, that the patient can remember as being related to the back pain. We tend to be very careful at this stage of the diagnosis because patients are quick to "attach" explanatory movements or events to the onset of their back pain. For instance they might be quick to say, "It was that exercise I was doing," "It was the way I bent over to pick up my glasses," or "It was the way I was holding my baby." If they incorrectly believe a certain movement caused the pain, they can develop disabling phobias about certain movements, which can be quite difficult to challenge even if they are clearly incorrect.

In sprain-strain there is usually local findings of tenderness over the area of discomfort, such as over the sacroiliac joint, over the paraspinal muscles (muscles on either side of the spine), and down to the upper part of the buttock area. The pain is made worse by bending forward or to the sides and, if more severe, may be associated with the type of muscle spasm that can actually be felt in the back muscles during the physical examination. It is important to remember that:

> **A sprain-strain is not a serious condition.**

A sprain-strain will heal naturally like any other injury. Research on animals has helped to identify more about the healing process of a sprain-strain to muscle. In these experiments a muscle (or muscles) are strained to the point of partial failure. At approximately twenty-four to forty-eight hours after the injury, a small amount of hemorrhage (bleeding in the muscle) was found where the muscle connects to the tendon. This bleeding was entirely gone at seven days after the strain. Also between twenty-four and forty-eight hours after the strain, microscopic examination showed inflammation in the area and a breakdown of the muscle fibers that were damaged. At forty-eight hours after the injury muscle function was already beginning to improve. More important, at seven days after the strain, function of the strained muscle had returned to normal levels. At that time it was also determined that an inelastic (i.e., not flexible) scar tissue was beginning develop to replace the damaged muscle fibers.

These findings can be generalized to humans in two important ways. First the natural healing time of a strain injury is actually quite rapid. It may be somewhat longer in the low back given the size and complexity of the muscles involved, but clinical experience supports the common finding of about six to eight weeks overall. Second is the aspect of scar tissue development. It has been found that healing tissue (or muscle) that has been immobilized has a tendency to produce scar tissue, which is nonfunctional, nonflexible, and has low strength. This type of scar tissue has been implicated in recurrent sprain-strain injuries. On the other hand quick reactivation of the injured muscles (within three to five days of injury) can help decrease the amount of scar tissue development and increase the strength and flexibility of the new muscle tissue that does develop. Don't worry if you have had a sprain-strain in the past and made the mistake (or your doctor did) of "resting" the injury. You are not doomed to recurrent back injuries. Getting on a regular strengthening and stretching program for your back and body can have the same positive effects.

In addition to the above physical factors in sprain-strain, one must remember that the pain is made worse by stress and anxiety. If this is occurring, it can create a vicious cycle of additional pain, which in turn causes more stress, tension, and pain. This may be one explanation for chronic, nonresolving back pain that began with a sprain-strain.

The natural history of a sprain-strain, once the activities that precipitated the injury have been corrected, is for healing to take place over a period of three to six weeks. The treatment is to *temporarily* stop or alter the activity that produces the complaint. In the very acute phase of the injury it may be helpful to use ice in the first twenty-four to forty-eight hours. This can be followed by the judicious use of moist heat, anti-inflammatory medication (such as salicylates), or a nonsteroidal anti-inflammatory. Occasionally for a severe sprain one or two days of rest in bed and the use of muscle relaxants for three or four days is appropriate, followed by the gradual resumption of activity. This is crucial to prevent deconditioning, stress, depression, fear of movement, and the chronic pain syndrome.

Additional formal treatment may sometimes be necessary, but not always. Besides the usual home remedies of short-term rest, ice followed by moist heat, and gentle return to activities, there is occasionally a place for a brief course of physical therapy. Physical therapy, in this setting, may often play the role of reactivating the patient, who may be more fearful of the pain and may have become somewhat deconditioned. The physical therapist will often guide the patient in a gentle stretching and exercise program. This should progress to a strengthening program, which will facilitate a return to normal functional activities. A home conditioning and strengthening program is often recommended to help prevent a susceptibility to future recurrences of lumbar sprains in deconditioned muscles.

The last phase of this treatment approach (reactivation and resumption of normal activities) is very important, as there is a small percentage of patients who initially sustain not much more than a sprain or strain of the low back and then go on to suffer chronic pain. The gradual resumption of activities shortly after the injury can help prevent this from occurring. Research has shown that the physical findings in *chronic back pain* patients are no more serious than in those patients who have had a back injury that resolves according to the natural healing time. This underscores the power of the "nonphysical" factors in the development of the chronic back pain problem.

Other reasons for the development of chronic pain likely include stress or other emotional factors, which we will discuss later. This may contribute to chronic changes in blood flow patterns to the back muscles, along with the anxiety over the pain, which will play a role in keeping the muscles perpetually in spasm.

Furthermore overtreatment with rest and passive therapy modalities (which is often done for sprain-strain injuries) will often lead to a deconditioned state in the muscles and a subsequent chronic pain syndrome. This fosters fear of activity and fear of further injury due to pain, which in turn will tend to keep the patient immobile, further exacerbating the deconditioned state. At this point patients can find themselves unintentionally getting comfortable in the sick role and actually being reinforced for being sick.

It should be kept in mind that this diagnosis is made on a clinical basis alone. There is no specific X ray, blood test, imaging study, or any other specific way of diagnosing a sprain or a strain. As a result of this, one thing to watch out for is the physician's or chiropractor's uneasiness in managing a sprain-strain problem. Since it is not a diagnosis that can be made in any definite sense, doctors will often tend to overrest, overrestrict, and overtreat patients for prolonged periods of time. This approach will actually compound the problem rather than help the patient improve.

A question often asked is: If an individual sustains a sprain or strain to his low back, does he or she have a higher likelihood of suffering recurrences of this problem or any tendency to develop a chronic low back pain problem? There is no clearcut scientific evidence to answer this question, although common sense and our clinical experience tells us that someone who remains in an overall well-conditioned state from a standpoint of flexibility and strength has a lower tendency and likelihood to have recurrent sprains and strains of the muscles. Generally an ongoing general exercise program is enough to keep the muscles better conditioned and less susceptible to these lumbar strains and sprains. Then, if an injury does occur, it is likely to resolve more quickly in the conditioned person. In some cases a more specific exercise program will be necessary, and the physical therapist can provide such a program.

It is critical to state that our clinical evidence shows that patients who tend to have chronic pain problems and recurrent lumbar sprain-strains often have significant nonphysical factors that appear to be playing a bigger role than the physiologic or physical factors of the muscles themselves. Patients who tend to focus on their body, are extremely fearful of pain, are being reinforced in the sick role, and have been given erroneous diagnoses would fall into this higher susceptibility category.

In summary, important factors in the treatment of sprain-strain problems include the following: (a) being extensively reassured about the likelihood of good resolution of symptoms due to natural healing; (b) limiting the amount of bed rest and gradually resuming activities; and (c) attending to the possibility that psychological factors may make you more susceptible to chronic pain and dealing with those, as is described later in the book.

Facet Syndrome

As you will recall from the anatomy chapter, the facet joints are located at the back of each vertebra and "attach" the vertebrae together. These are the joints, like the joints in your fingers, that connect the bones of the spine together and allow them to move with reference to one another.

In "facet syndrome" there is an inflammation of one or more facet joints. This inflammation can produce referred pain, or pain that is perceived someplace other than where it is being caused (e.g., in your buttock or on the outside of your thigh, down usually as far as your knee but no farther). A facet syndrome is usually diagnosed, like a sprain-strain, based on a clinical presentation. Often there is a localized area of tenderness, 1 to 1½ inches to the side of the midpoint of the spine in the lower back. Pressure in this specific area will cause discomfort in this region, plus sometimes farther down into the buttock or thigh area. The pain is usually made worse by certain activities, such as extending, bending forward, twisting to one side or the other, and standing on one leg.

Facet syndrome is an uncommon occurrence and is not serious. It can be painful but will usually resolve over a period of two to three weeks, and the treatment is the same as for a sprain-strain. In rare instances where it becomes chronic (doesn't go away within two to three weeks), it can occasionally be treated effectively by a local injection of anti-inflammatory and anesthetic medication into the irritated joint. An appropriate exercise program should also be part of this treatment program.

Arthritis of the Spine

Arthritis is a general term that means inflammation of a joint or joints. It can be seen in any joint in the body, including those of the spine. There are many different causes and types of arthritis, some a natural part of aging, with no symptoms, and others quite severe in terms of pain and deformation. Unfortunately the term has become more associated with the crippling conditions than it has with the normal aging process. As such this is an extremely frightening diagnosis to most patients, though it doesn't have to be so. Arthritis of the spine often occurs as part of the natural aging process.

Arthritis of the spine is most often not associated with any symptoms.

The diagnosis is frequently given based solely on X ray or imaging findings of bone spurs, which often play no role in someone's pain. True arthritis in the spine is a disorder called ankylosing spondylitis (to be discussed later), which is associated with more severe inflammation and stiffening of the spine. Ankylosing spondylitis is quite rare and is usually diagnosed and treated by rheumatology specialists.

In reality the term *arthritis* should rarely be used in describing joint changes in the spine. It often conjures up an image in many people's minds of a crippling condition remembered from a childhood experience of seeing an old aunt or grandmother with gnarled fingers or a crooked spine. Its use should be restricted to those very rare instances in conditions such as ankylosing spondylitis or rheumatoid arthritis.

Rheumatoid Arthritis (Ankylosing Spondylitis)

When you think of the most crippling aspects of the general condition of arthritis, you're picturing rheumatoid arthritis—it usually occurs in various joints of the body and rarely in the spine. If it does occur in the spine, it is diagnosed by X-ray findings of joint deformity and blood tests to detect the "rheumatoid factor." It is generally treated with anti-inflammatory medications, gentle exercises, injections of special medications, and appropriate braces. This condition is progressive, and treatment is generally aimed at improving the quality of life to the highest possible level.

Ankylosing spondylitis, which means "an inflammation and stiffening" of the spine, is a form of rheumatoid arthritis involving the joints of the spine, occurring primarily in young males. It is diagnosed by appropriate blood tests and occasionally X rays. This condition, which rarely results in significant disability, can frequently be treated quite effectively with a regular exercise program (although it might be painful), medications, and sometimes a brace.

Degenerative Disc Disease

Similar to arthritis of the spine, degenerative disc disease is not a true "disease" in most instances. Rather it is simply a description of a normal wear-and-tear process whereby the soft central portion of the disc loses its water content and begins to dry up. This process usually starts at about the age of twenty years old and proceeds throughout life. On rare occasions this condition can lead to a "mechanical type" of low back pain in which strenuous physical activity in a person who is not adequately conditioned will cause back pain.

Degenerative disc disease, if it does cause symptoms, is treated with an appropriate exercise program, the use of correct spinal mechanics, and occasionally a mild anti-inflammatory medication. It virtually never requires any type of surgical treatment.

In summary, *degenerative disc disease* is a scary term for something that happens to every human being on the face of the planet! To ease your fears, it is useful to think of it as being similar to male-pattern baldness. Both of these conditions are not "diseases" in a true sense at all, but rather are associated with those unfortunate people who continue to get older. (Who *doesn't* fall into that group?)

Arachnoiditis

Arachnoiditis is an inflammation or scarring of the connective tissues (the spinal arachnoid) around the spinal nerve roots. *Arachnoid* literally means "like a cobweb" and this is how the condition looks on imaging studies. The most common cause of arachnoiditis is surgery. The symptoms are pain, numbness, and tingling in the lower extremities. The symptoms are unfortunately not very responsive to such treatments as usual pain medicines or physical therapy. On rare occasions a cortisone injection can be temporarily beneficial. In severe cases the use of a spinal cord stimulator may be useful.

Arachnoiditis does not always preclude surgery provided there are other causes for the ongoing pain. Arachnoiditis itself cannot be treated by surgery, and there is always the risk that surgery will make the arachnoiditis worse.

Spondylolisthesis and Spondylolysis

Spondylolisthesis, which means "slipping vertebrae," refers to a condition in which one vertebra "slips" (has a forward displacement) over another. This can be caused by a stress fracture or a crack in part of the vertebral body between two connecting joints, which is termed a *spondylolysis*. The fracture can result from trauma, usually over a period of time during the teenage years. It can cause pain in the low back and occasionally sciatic pain if the nerve roots are involved.

Spondylolisthesis is seen with frequency in gymnasts, ballet dancers, and football players, as it is often caused by the trauma of hyperextension repeated over several times. Usually no one incident will cause the fracture, but repeated episodes result in an actual break. Initially the crack is so fine that it will not be visible on a regular X ray. Therefore if spondylolysis is suspected, it is appropriate to have a bone scan, which can detect very fine "cracks" in the vertebrae (this will be discussed in chapter 7). A common possible indicator of this condition would be a backache in a young person for more than one or two weeks. If the fracture can be diagnosed at the time it occurs (usually between the ages of thirteen and sixteen years old), it can be treated very effectively with complete resolution. If it goes unrecognized, it can cause back-pain problems in later life.

Treatment, whether in childhood or in adulthood, includes an appropriate brace for a period of about four months, which is worn during the day, and a temporary limitation of activities. This will allow a high percentage of healing to take place, at the conclusion of which the person's spine will often return to a "normal" state. In severe cases of "slipping" (spondylolisthesis) a spinal fusion surgery may be necessary.

The other common type of spondylolisthesis is termed *degenerative spondylolisthesis* and is caused by wear-and-tear changes in the facet joint or connecting joints of the lower back due to a variety of different factors. The most common site is usually between the fourth and fifth lumbar vertebrae, with the former slipping forward on the latter. In diagnostic terms all types of spondylolisthesis are graded, I–IV, with "I" being the least amount of "slippage" and "IV" being the greatest.

Spina Bifida Occulta

Spina bifida occulta is simply a defect in the lamina, or the back part of the vertebral body. This occurs due to a failure of formation during fetal development within the uterus. It is present in approximately 8 percent of the population and is not a cause of low back pain.

Scoliosis

Scoliosis is a term used to describe a curvature of the spine. It has several different varieties, but in essence it is an unusual cause of low back pain in people under forty years old unless it is quite severe.

> **Mild curvatures of the spine are quite common, need no specific treatment, and are not associated with an increased frequency of low back pain.**

The key element with respect to scoliosis is whether or not it is progressive (curving more and more). A very small percentage of scoliosis in the lower back progresses and needs to be treated appropriately. In the vast majority of cases, however, these are incidental findings and need no specific treatment. You should be warned that this diagnosis is commonly mislabeled and given as a cause for back pain with recommendations for extensive treatment to straighten out the spine. Curves under 20 degrees, which represent the great majority of scoliosis seen clinically, need no treatment and are not known to be causes of pain.

Osteoarthritis
Osteoarthritis, which means "inflammation of a bony joint" is frequently seen in the hip as a cause of sciatic-type pain in the elderly population. It is usually diagnosed, if thought of by the doctor, from an appropriate X ray of the hips and pelvis. It involves a wear-and-tear type of arthritis, or a wearing out of the cover of the bones of the hip joint (a ball-and-socket-type joint).

Bursitis
Bursitis is an inflammation of the bursa, which is a space between a tendon and the bone or between two tendons. The most common type of bursitis that coexists with low back pain is bursitis of the hip. This is sometimes called trochanteric

bursitis and can cause pain in the buttock, or the outer or back of the thigh. This condition is often confused with sciatica.

Bursitis is diagnosed based on the patient's history and what the physician finds during a physical examination. There is no specific X-ray test, imaging study, or blood test to make this diagnosis.

The treatment for this type of bursitis is stretching exercises, anti-inflammatory medication, and the temporary cessation of those activities that appear to precipitate the pain. Occasionally an injection of an anti-inflammatory and anesthetic medicine into the area of discomfort can be helpful.

Osteomyelitis

Osteomyelitis is an infection in the vertebrae or bones of the spine. It rarely occurs and is manifested by pain at rest, loss of weight, and occasionally fever. It is detected on a number of diagnostic tests including abnormal blood findings and is treated with a brace and appropriate antibiotics for a period of three to six weeks. It usually resolves without the need for surgery.

Discitis

Discitis is a rare condition and means literally "inflammation of the disc." Although the exact cause is not clear, it is thought to occur due to a bacterial or viral infection in the disc space. This causes inflammation and pain. Although it can occur in people of all ages, it is more common in those under twenty years of age, persons with diabetes, or other individuals with immune system problems.

It is appropriately treated by antibiotics if bacteria is the cause. In children the treatment is usually a brace.

Transitional Vertebrae

Transitional vertebrae, like spina bifida occulta and minimal degrees of scoliosis, is frequently seen on X rays and is not associated with increased incidence of low back pain. This condition is found at the base of the lumbar spine where it connects to the sacrum. It can represent either one extra lumbar vertebrae or one less lumbar vertebrae.

Coccydynia

Coccydynia means "pain in the coccyx." It is a condition of pain in the bone at the very lower base of the spine known as the coccyx. It is often a result of trauma, usually from a direct fall upon the buttocks, and results in a persistence of pain just above the rectal area. The pain is usually very localized and the region is tender to touch.

Treatment usually consists of avoidance of sitting on hard surfaces or direct contact with the seat. Often the use of a donutlike seat cushion is recommended. Furthermore anti-inflammatory medication and occasional local injection of anesthetics and steroids are indicated in more refractory cases. There is also some recent research that suggests that a special type of biofeedback to teach the person to relax secondary local muscle spasm can be helpful.

Surgery may be considered as a last resort in more chronic and severe cases that have not responded to any other interventions. However, certainly psychological evaluation should precede any surgical interventions in patients with chronic, severe coccydynia, as emotional factors often impact this condition. Also, it should be known that surgery is not consistently found to be successful in this disorder.

Other Spinal Fractures

Spinal fractures are almost always seen in one of two circumstances. They sometimes occur in the younger population following a severe trauma, such as a motor vehicle accident or a fall. And they also include compression fractures, which often cause a pie-shaped appearance to the vertebral body on the X ray. These are seen in association with weakening of the bone due to an underlying disease process, which might be either osteoporosis, as seen most commonly in postmenopausal females, or in patients in whom cancer has spread to the spinal column. A person over forty years old who develops back pain that is not associated with activity, that is so severe that it can wake him or her from sleep, and that does not resolve within a period of a week or two needs to be evaluated by a physician familiar with spine disorders, as these symptoms might represent a more serious problem.

Osteoporosis

As mentioned above, a common form of spinal fracture is associated with osteoporosis in the elderly female population. These fractures rarely cause significant deformity. The pain associated with these fractures is usually minimal and may last three to six weeks after the onset. The treatment usually consists of altered activity, mild analgesics, and the occasional use of an appropriate brace or corset.

An internist or gynecologist should evaluate and treat the underlying condition of osteoporosis that weakened the bone and caused the fracture. Taking supplemental calcium can help prevent this condition. The question of whether or not estrogen therapy should be instituted around the time of menopause is controversial and needs to be discussed with the internist or gynecologist.

Most patients with osteoporotic compression fractures return to normal functioning with minimal residual pain. Traumatic compression fractures, as well, in younger patients often resolve without any long-term pain or deformities. This condition is treated appropriately with painkillers and bracing, often for approximately six weeks.

Back Problems with Pregnancy

Back pain occurs frequently in pregnancy and usually resolves after delivery with no long-term changes in function or residual pain. The cause of back pain in pregnancy remains somewhat controversial. Common reasons include the mechanical factors of increased abdominal girth and the weight of the fetus putting excessive strain on the back while weakening the abdominal muscles and lessening the support to the spine. Furthermore hormonal changes during pregnancy can lead to relaxation of the ligaments that support the low back and pelvis, causing back pain.

A good exercise program with attention to proper mechanics of the spine should help reduce the incidents and/or intensity of back pain during pregnancy.

Idiopathic Back Pain

Idiopathic back pain is defined as back pain without a well-known cause, which, as previously stated, may describe a great majority of the back pain that we presently see. This diagnosis has been used to describe "stress-related back pain" or "non-specific mechanical low back pain." These diagnoses will be discussed later.

Subluxation

Subluxation is a term frequently used by chiropractors and osteopaths to explain the underlying reason for low back pain. Literally this would mean the partial loss of continuity between two joint surfaces (a dislocation is a total loss of continuity between two joint surfaces, such as in a dislocation of the shoulder). In fact subluxations relative to the joints of the lower back, if they occur, have not been demonstrated with certainty on standard X rays or CT scans. Whether or not subluxations actually occur as a cause of back pain is a point of controversy among physicians treating spinal disorders.

Chiropractors often use the term *subluxation* to indicate a restriction in a certain joint, with some type of limitation of movement that can be fixed with manipulation. The manipulation is purported to realign the "subluxed," or restricted, joint.

Caution should be used with this diagnosis, as chiropractors and other health care practitioners frequently recommend extensive, long-term treatment to address this problem, which is often not clearly responsible for the pain. In any case any long-term treatment approach has many counterproductive sides, such as creating a dependency of the patient on the health care practitioner and likely facilitating several psychological factors that initiate and contribute to chronic pain syndromes.

Research has shown there may be a role for spinal manipulation in acute low back pain as a treatment that may be cost-effective and valuable in the first couple of months. This has

been supported by several articles in the medical literature in
the past few years.

Lumbar Spinal Stenosis

Lumbar stenosis means a "narrowing" of the bony spinal canal and causes a compression or "pinching" of the nerves passing through the area going to the buttocks and lower
extremities. The stenosis can occur for many reasons, including such things as disc bulges, wear-and-tear changes leading to
bone spurs, or congenital narrowing (from birth). Whatever
the cause, the end result is that the spinal canal through which
the nerves pass is somehow made smaller.

Lumbar stenosis most typically limits the ability to walk distances or at a fast pace. People will often lean forward at the
waist to relieve the pain as they walk. These patients will often
report that walking in a grocery store while leaning on the cart
will decrease symptoms. They will also sit down for a short
period of time or stoop until the symptoms subside. The activities that decrease pain, such as leaning and sitting, help open
the spinal canal more and therefore temporarily decrease the
pressure on the nerves.

The diagnosis of lumbar stenosis is made from the history
obtained from the patient, combined with the absence of other
causes that limit walking ability (such as hardening of the arter-
ies, arthritis of the hips, and problems in the knees or ankles).
The diagnosis is confirmed by either an MRI, CT scan, or
CT-myelogram. Due to the aging changes (degenerative), this
diagnosis is rather common in the elderly population over
sixty-five. With the increase in this proportion of our population, the diagnosis is being made more frequently each passing
year.

Although the condition is usually progressive, it does not
lead to paralysis, shortening of life, or loss of life. Its most
serious consequences are at times the rather significant limitations of functional capacity. The natural history is one of slow
progression in perhaps 50 percent of the patients.

The treatment consists of three phases. First is a "flexion"
exercise program, combined with the short-term use of nonste-

roidal anti-inflammatory medication. Second is a "low-volume" epidural injection of anti-inflammatory medication into the space surrounding the spinal nerves, which may alleviate the condition for a period of time. And the third and most definitive form of treatment is a surgical widening of the spinal canal via a laminectomy (removal of the lamina), which in effect gives the nerves more room.

Fibromyalgia

Fibromyalgia is a diagnosis often made in patients suffering with chronic low back pain. Characteristics include sleep disturbance, multiple tender points, fatigue, diffuse pain, and limitations of activity. Associated symptoms are numerous and can include irritable bowel syndrome, chronic headaches, chest pain, memory impairment, anxiety, and depression, among others. There are several terms that have been used to describe this complex pain problem, including fibrositis, myofascial pain syndrome, and tension myalgia, just to mention a few. The diagnosis has been written about extensively in the medical literature, although there continues to be no clear understanding of the cause or cure.

Current treatment programs generally use anti-inflammatory medications to help with the pain, antidepressant medicines for their effect on sleep and depression, and a gradual increase in exercise and activity.

This is one diagnostic label, in our experience, that can lead to a variety of treatments over a long period of time without any significant benefit. It does appear that there may be significant psychological and emotional issues that are part of fibromyalgia. Whether these are related to the cause or are in reaction to the problem is unknown. A recent review of the research literature concluded, "When all available psychological research is considered, it is apparent that psychological disturbance is associated with FS (Fibromyalgia Syndrome). . . . Furthermore, it is not clear that psychological disturbance can predict a specific chronic pain syndrome such as FS or whether psychological disturbance is the general result of experiencing chronic pain."

Our advice to patients with the diagnosis is to keep the treatment simple, straightforward, and time-limited. This might include a brief trial of anti-inflammatory medicines and antidepressant medicines, and a reasonable exercise program with gradual resumption of normal activities. Although there are many self-help groups nationally for fibromyalgia, we have found that these tend to make patients worse. They often focus on the search for a cure and continuance of the sick role. In addition, if you have been diagnosed with fibromyalgia, it will be imperative to investigate psychological and emotional factors that may be making your symptoms worse. The following two diagnoses are similar to fibromyalgia but have a greater emphasis on emotional factors.

Tension Myalgia Syndrome

This diagnosis and the one following (stress-related back pain) are ones that you will not hear within traditional medical circles. As discussed at the beginning of the chapter, we feel these conditions are quite common. We also believe that an incorrect structural diagnosis is often given when actually one of these two diagnoses is accurate.

The Mayo Clinic has used and researched the diagnosis of tension myalgia syndrome for over forty years. In this term *myalgia* refers to the widespread muscle pain that is characteristic in this condition. The word *tension* refers to two states: physical and emotional. Physical tension applies to the muscles being "in spasm" or "tight," possibly resulting from postural stressors, poor body mechanics, varying degrees of trauma such as is seen in sprain-strains, or nonrestorative sleep. The second component of the word *tension* is the psychological or emotional tension associated with the condition. In our clinical experience the latter of these tension factors appears to be quite significant.

Symptoms of tension myalgia syndrome are very similar to fibromyalgia, if not identical. They include generalized aches and pain (either regional or generalized), tender points, nonrestorative sleep, fatigue, type A personality (to be discussed later), and a lack of other conditions that might explain the symptoms.

The focus of recommended treatment for this disorder by the Mayo Clinic is quite similar to the treatment recommended by most rheumatologists for the treatment of fibromyalgia. This includes education and reassurance that the condition is not serious, physical therapy and conditioning aimed at returning to normal function, certain medications, relaxation training, as well as psychological pain management to help deal with the emotional or psychological stressors considered to be playing a role. The medications used might often include antidepressants in low doses, which can assist the individual in normalizing sleep patterns. Furthermore recommendations are given for an ongoing home exercise program including stretching, strengthening, and aerobic exercises.

Many medical professionals treating these conditions (fibromyalgia and tension myalgia syndrome) recommend multiple rest periods and significant limitations on the amount of exercise and overall physical activities, as guided by the patient's levels of pain and fatigue. It has been our experience that these recommended activity restrictions and subsequently self-imposed limitations have often resulted in an unnecessary contribution to pain, functional limitation, and deconditioning. This will be discussed in greater detail in later chapters.

It is the opinion of the authors of this book that emotions and various psychological stressors often referred to as tension play a large role in this type of chronic back pain.

Stress-Related Back Pain

This diagnosis takes the idea of psychological and emotional factors in back pain one step farther in its orientation that these are of absolute primary influence. The diagnosis of stress-related back pain is a "psychosomatic" or "psychophysiological" one. This means that psychological factors either initiated or are maintaining the symptoms, or both. A psychophysiological illness is any illness in which physical symptoms are thought to be the direct result of psychological or emotional factors. Individuals most often focus on the physical problem to the exclusion of emotional issues. However, these conditions are not imaginary. There are real physical problems, which are being impacted upon by emotional factors.

The diagnosis of stress-related back pain is often made by history and physical exam, which should easily be able to rule out the more serious structural causes of back pain in a great majority of patients. The characteristics of stress-related back pain are essentially the same as in tension myalgia syndrome and fibromyalgia. These include diffuse muscle ache, sleep disturbances, and fatigue, among others.

Dr. John Sarno, a physician and professor of physical medicine and rehabilitation at New York University, has recently popularized the idea of stress-related back pain, although the concept can be traced to as early as the 1820s. For instance in his book *From Paralysis to Fatigue,* Dr. Edward Shorter traces the history of psychosomatic illness in modern times, including stress-related back pain. The diagnosis of "spinal irritation" was coined in the 1820s and was prevalent until about the 1890s.

As Dr. Shorter quotes from a doctor writing on the subject in 1829,

> The lower extremities become the seat of various morbid sensations, spasms, et cetera, for the most part resembling those which have been described in the upper limbs. The patients also complain of a sense of insecurity or instability in walking; their knees totter and feel scarcely able to support the weight of the body. . . . This irritation, or subacute inflammatory state [meaning no inflammation was demonstrated] of the spinal marrow is not necessarily connected with any deformity of the spine or disease in the vertebrae.

This diagnosis spread greatly throughout the world from this point on. Interestingly Dr. Shorter makes the point that doctors and patients of the era began to believe firmly in the diagnosis even though there was no demonstrable pathology. This diagnosis led to serious disease attribution by patients and helped doctors justify their treatments (a process similar to what occurs today). Dr. Shorter points out that the physicians of the day would implant the disease attribution in the patient's head, increase fear that serious disease existed, and recommend "rigid maintenance of the horizontal position." He continues, in referring to the treatment of a patient by saying that, "Obeying this recommendation, which accords with her own instincts, the unfortunate maiden stretches herself supine upon the bed or sofa, and vegetates many a weary month in slothful languor."

The diagnosis remained fairly prevalent until the early 1900s. Dr. Shorter points out that the diagnosis served the doctors' needs in terms of remaining competitive with other medical clinics by "medicalizing" the patients' ill-defined subjective complaints. Also it served the patients' needs by providing a "face-saving" medical diagnosis rather than having to look at possible psychological and emotional factors. Patients would always feel more comfortable with the "spinal irritation" diagnosis than with looking to emotions.

Although the foregoing has been a rather long digression into history, we feel it is helpful in understanding current medical approaches to back pain.

> **Many doctors continue to look primarily for structural "explanations" for back pain, convince their patient that the "finding" is the cause of the pain, implant fear in the patient, and then recommend "justifiable" treatment.**

In returning to Dr. Sarno's conceptualization of stress-related back pain, one can see the similarities with that of "spinal irritation" (and even with fibromyalgia and tension myalgia syndrome). The important difference is that Dr. Sarno places the causative factors for the pain squarely in the psychological and emotional realm. Doctors treating spinal irritation did not, and even if they did, it was not discussed openly with their patients. Rather, placebo treatment (a treatment that the patient believes in but that actually has no curative power) was used. Related to this, Dr. Sarno believes that a majority of back-pain cases are being treated by the medical community with "organic" approaches when the pain is actually stress related. This pattern is very similar to spinal irritation, discussed above.

Patients with stress-related back pain show characteristic tender points, and their history of onset is often quite variable. The pain may start with an identifiable incident, or it may start insidiously. Often we will see the pain start with an incident such as a lumbar sprain-strain, only to have it continue as the result of emotional factors long after the injury has healed.

Dr. Sarno believes that stress-related back pain is not due to mechanical factors but has more to do with people's feelings and personalities. Key emotions are anger and anxiety. In addition he describes people who are likely to get stress-related back pain as being similar to the type A personality, including a strong inner drive to succeed, having a great sense of responsibility, being self-motivated and disciplined, being their own severest critics, and being perfectionistic and compulsive. These personality characteristics interact with stressful life situations to cause the back pain. He points out that the source of psychological and emotional tension is not always obvious.

This theory explains a mechanism whereby emotional tension is pushed out of awareness by the mind into the unconscious. This unconscious tension causes changes in the body's nervous system. These changes include constriction in blood vessels and reduction of blood flow to the various soft tissues, including muscles, tendons, ligaments, and nerves in the back. This causes a decrease in oxygen to the area as well as a buildup of biochemical waste products in the muscles. In turn this results in muscle tension, spasm, and pain experienced by the patient.

Even at this point the cycle is not complete. The pain leads to the patient becoming unnecessarily limited in many functions of daily life, as well as leisure activities. This decrease in activities is due to the patient's being afraid of the pain as well as admonition from doctors making a structural diagnosis, which results in more pain, more fear, and more deconditioning (sound similar to spinal irritation?).

His approach to patients with this diagnosis is one of emphasizing the psychological and emotional factors as causative and reassuring the patient as to the importance of a return to full physical functioning. Again, this is where Dr. Sarno's approach differs from what happened with spinal irritation and the way most physicians manage patients with these symptoms. Once the diagnosis of stress-related back pain is made, the treatment is similar to that for tension myalgia, with the additional strong recommendation to "think psychological, not physical" when the pain occurs.

More concepts associated with this condition will be discussed further throughout this book.

The Deconditioning Syndrome
Throughout this book you will see much mention of the deconditioning or deactivation syndrome. This is a condition that results from a person "resting" his or her back pain by doing such things as stopping exercise and engaging in more bed rest and reclining. Physical inactivity results in a progressive decrease in the size, strength, and flexibility of muscles and ligaments. In addition it leads to diminished cardiovascular and muscular endurance. This is the worst possible thing a person with back pain could do.

The deconditioning syndrome has also been termed the disuse syndrome, referring to how it develops. Research has documented that excessive rest and disuse have negative effects on virtually every body system. The exact effects of disuse will be discussed further in the aggressive conditioning chapter.

The deconditioning syndrome can occur either beginning with or in conjunction with virtually any of the above-mentioned diagnoses. The problem is that if the person is resting his or her back pain, the original injury will often heal (such as in a sprain-strain), but the deconditioning syndrome will continue to cause back pain. This needs to be treated with aggressive reconditioning and "working through" the pain.

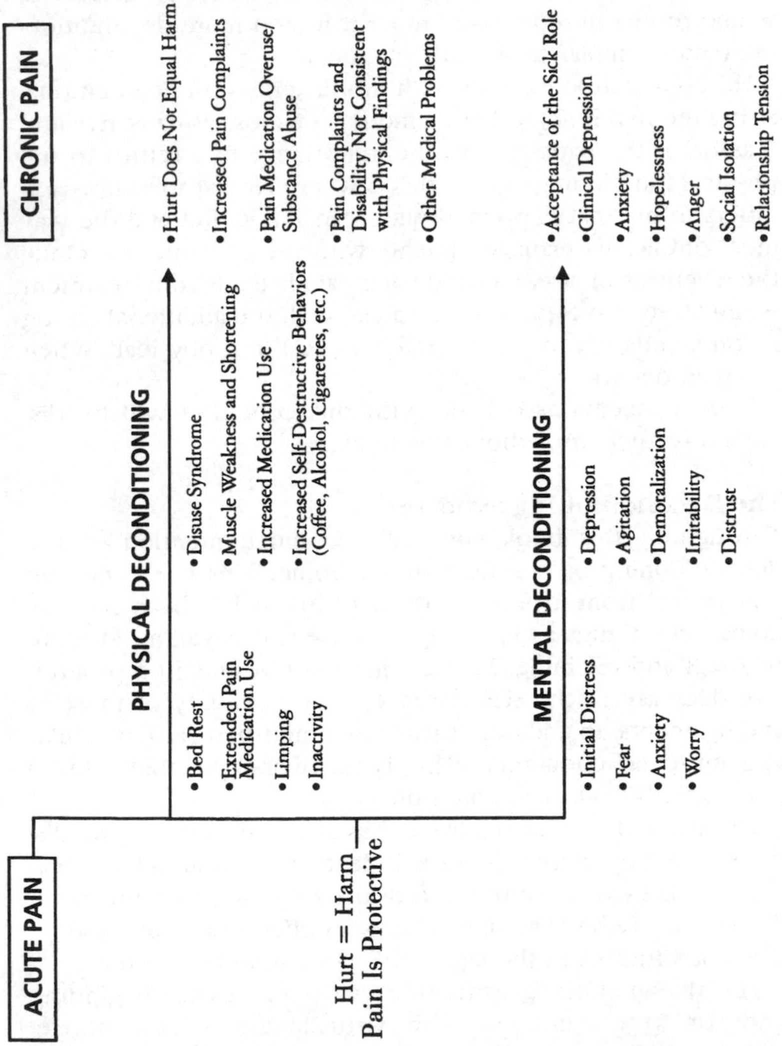

Figure 6-1. Development of chronic back pain due to physical and mental deconditioning. Adapted from Dr. Robert Gatchel, 1991. Illustration provided courtesy of Century City Hospital, Los Angeles.

Chronic Back-Pain Syndrome

As discussed previously, *chronic pain* is defined as pain that goes beyond the point of tissue healing or an approximate time span of three to six months. The *chronic back-pain syndrome* is a group of symptoms that can occur as a result of chronic back pain. The process by which these other symptoms occur has been generally termed physical and mental deconditioning by Drs. Robert Gatchel and Tom Mayer. This is a process whereby the individual shows more and more symptoms over time as the pain continues. The stages of development of physical and mental deconditioning leading to a chronic pain syndrome can be seen in figure 6-1.

> **By the time the chronic back-pain syndrome is fully developed, many (or most) of the symptoms are not related to the original pain problem but rather due to such things as the disuse syndrome, pain medication overuse, depression and anxiety, and social isolation, among others.**

The Failed-Back-Surgery Syndrome

The failed-back-surgery syndrome is unfortunately all too common. The syndrome is similar to the chronic back-pain syndrome discussed above, except that it follows some type of spine surgery (e.g., lumbar discectomy, decompressions, and fusions). The syndrome presents as a cluster of symptoms including pain, as well as physical and mental dysfunction.

Failed-back-surgery syndrome occurs for a variety of reasons. These include such things as early infection after surgery, a spine fusion at the wrong level, psychological distress, inadequate reconditioning after surgery, a failed fusion (pseudoarthrosis), or some other physical problem (stenosis, disc degeneration, arachnoiditis, instability near the fusion, etc.).

Many of these conditions have been discussed previously in this chapter.

Treatment for the failed-back-surgery syndrome virtually never includes more surgery, but instead involves a conservative, noninvasive approach such as that used in the chronic back-pain syndrome. The most prudent approach is a multidisciplinary pain or functional restoration program. Many controversial treatment measures have been developed for the failed-back-surgery syndrome, and these are discussed in chapter 10.

CHAPTER 7

DIAGNOSTIC TESTING

By far the most important and useful diagnostic test with respect to low back pain is a complete and thorough history taken by your doctor in a face-to-face interview. In most instances a well-trained spinal physician should be able to have a relatively clear idea of what is causing your back problem after your history has been taken. The physical examination should be basically to confirm the diagnostic impression based on the history, and in most instances will do so. One of the primary problems in history taking with regard to patients with low back pain is that the physician may be too focused on the back pain itself to the exclusion of social and emotional factors. This includes such things as how the pain influences the patient's day-to-day life, what anxieties and fears it is producing, and how it interferes with the patient's social adaptations and overall functional capacity. If the doctor focuses only on mechanical-structural diagnostic possibilities, the diagnosis and treatment will often be incorrect.

Unfortunately many of the advances in technology over the past two decades have allowed doctors to give the false impression that they need to rely less on a good history and physical examination and can simply proceed to diagnostic testing for the "answer" to the low back pain. Patients are usually more than willing to accept this approach because they tend to believe that the more high-tech the machine, the more accurate it is. Nothing could be farther from the truth. These tests are very sensitive and allow us to see normal wear-and-tear changes present in the spine that are not abnormal in any way and may be seen in a person with no symptoms. Given this fact, it is even more crucial than ever that the history be detailed and appropriate so that the physician can identify which of those changes seen on X ray are clinically significant and which are not.

QUESTIONS TO ASK ABOUT THE TEST

As we have discussed previously, you should feel that you are in a partnership with your doctor or health care provider. Approaching the recommendation for diagnostic testing should be no different. The following questions are useful to ask of your doctor if testing has been recommended:

- What is the test and what does it show?
- Why is it performed and why am I being advised to have it?
- What can I expect before, during, and after the test?
- What does it mean if the test is "positive" or "negative"?

These few questions should give you a very good idea about the testing. Throughout the diagnostic phase of your doctor's evaluation of your pain, you should keep in mind:

The results of any diagnostic test without reference to the whole person are of no value and can be counterproductive.

With that in mind we will proceed with an explanation of each diagnostic test, attempting to answer the above questions.

DIAGNOSTIC TESTING IN BACK PAIN

Plain X Rays

An X ray uses a low level of radiation in order to view the bones of the spine. In the X ray, radiation is passed through the specific body area and casts an image on a piece of film. The X-ray picture is called a radiograph. The radiation exposure is very small, being less than the amount you would receive on an airplane flight from Los Angeles to New York.

When this test is used in regard to back pain, it allows us to see the bones comprising the lumbar spine, sacroiliac joint, and pelvis. We can identify whether or not there are changes associated with normal aging, fractures, and the overall alignment of the spine (scoliosis, etc). The test is appropriate in those persons whose lower back pain has not resolved over the initial two to three weeks of conservative treatment and/or in a person who has nonactivity-related back pain or pain that awakens him or her at night.

It should *not* routinely be used on a person's first visit to the doctor for back pain unless there are very clear reasons (e.g., trauma). At the stage of the first visit it is not worth doing and is not cost-effective. It has been shown in recent research studies that in only 19 percent of cases are there meaningful data obtained from X rays done on the first visit for low back pain. Again, in cases where there is a significant history of trauma, obtaining X rays at the time of the first visit is reasonable in order to rule out fractures. Otherwise the history and physical examination should be key elements of the first doctor visit.

The X-ray process is very simple and painless. When possible, the person performing the tests should offer to allow you to cover the genital areas with a lead shield if you wish. Except for women in the first three months of pregnancy, X rays are a safe procedure and are without side effects.

So-called positive, or abnormal, findings on the X ray of the spine in most instances mean nothing. In fact they may not be related in any sense to the low back pain you are experiencing, but are simply a reflection of normal aging changes in the spine. Positive findings that might relate to your back pain include such conditions as a fracture, severe degeneration, or significant scoliosis.

If the tests are negative, patients will often ask, "Why do I have pain?" This is because the great majority of painful conditions of the back emanate from the soft tissues of the spine, the muscles, the joint capsules, the tendons, the ligaments, and the discs. None of these structures are imaged or visualized on a plain X ray.

The MRI (Magnetic Resonance Imaging)

An MRI, which stands for *"magnetic resonance imaging,"* is a relatively new imaging study. It utilizes a strong magnetic field, radio waves, and a computer to obtain a picture of many structures of the spine. MRI does not use X-ray exposure or require exposure to radiation. It will show your doctor the discs, nerves, muscles, and ligaments, as well as the bones that are visualized on plain X ray. Thus it gives far more information than plain X ray. No definitive risks have yet been identified with the performance of an MRI test; however, the test is not at this time known to be totally safe for women in the early stages of pregnancy. It is also not used on patients with pacemakers.

We feel MRIs are generally appropriate if the patient is a possible surgical candidate, has not responded to appropriate conservative management over a period of six to eight weeks, or is possibly suffering from an infection or tumor of the spine. These criteria are currently being developed by national experts and will become more customary over the next year.

This test is so sensitive that it allows us to image very subtle aging changes in the spine that are normal in a large percentage of the population who have no symptoms (especially in the age group over thirty-five or forty). In these cases the identified "abnormalities" are not responsible for the patient's symptoms. In fact even if they are responsible for the pain, in a great majority of instances the identification of these changes does not impact the recommended treatment for the condition.

Unfortunately MRI tests are frequently misused and overused by physicians for a number of reasons. First, doctors recommend MRI tests to allay their anxiety about diagnosing their patient. Physicians who treat a lot of back pain should generally be comfortable with their diagnosis based on the history and physical examination. Those who are less confident will order an MRI on every single patient; this is clearly inappropriate.

Second, many practitioners will order an MRI to avoid a lawsuit in the case of "missed diagnoses." This is not good practice in medicine and leads to excessive costs for the patient as well as instilling fear that something "terrible" must be wrong.

Third, and possibly most unfortunate, is the routine ordering of MRIs as a justification for what may be unnecessary spine surgery. The results of an "abnormal" MRI can also be used to justify ongoing treatment and/or prolongation of disability following work injuries, automobile accidents, slip-and-fall cases, etc. In this scenario the "abnormal" findings (which are actually normal) are used to justify treatments that are generally doomed to fail.

The MRI procedure is very safe and virtually without side effects. There is no special preparation prior to the testing. You will be placed on a scanning table, which slides into the giant magnet, which is shaped like a large tube. About 20 percent of the patients who undergo the procedure find being in the "tube" uncomfortable due to feelings of claustrophobia. If you think you might fall into this category, arrangements can be made to take a sedative. Because of this many of the newer facilities have developed the use of prism glasses, earphones so that one can listen to music, and even large television screens for purposes of distraction. All of these things can help lessen the anxiety associated with being in this confined space.

Once in the tube, you will hear several noises including a humming sound, a thump when the radio waves are turned on and off, and other machine noises. The most difficult part of the test for people with back pain is lying still for an extended period of time (forty-five to sixty minutes). Occasionally doctors will order an MRI with "an enhancement agent." This is simply a fluid injected into your arm or leg. The enhancement agent can help make the MRI picture clearer, especially in patients who have had prior surgery.

It should be noted that there are open machines that are less claustrophobic; however, the resolution and the quality of the picture suffer greatly. If at all possible, if an MRI is to be done, one should attempt to have it done in the best machine possible with the largest magnet.

As with all other tests, if an MRI shows anything, the results are meaningless unless this information is integrated into the other findings.

If the MRI reveals essentially "normal" findings, patients will often ask, "Why do I have pain?" For reasons that medicine does not yet fully understand, pain can come from sources we are not able to identify, even on MRI. Such things include pain from an inflammation, sprain-strain in the muscle-ligament complex, and stress-related back pain.

The CT Scan

CT scan stands for "computerized tomography" (it is also referred to as a CAT scan, which is "computerized axial tomography"). These words reflect the nature of the test. *Computerized* means that a very sophisticated computer is required to make the final picture. *Tomography* comes from the Greek words *tomos* (which means a "slice" or "section") and *graphia* (which means "recording"). Thus a CT scan is the computerized recording of a slice or section of the body.

The CT scanner uses X ray to produce images that the computer organizes into many thin "slices" or cross-sections of the body. As such there is a moderate amount of radiation exposure, which is greater than plain X ray but still well within the safe range. The scans that are produced allow for excellent viewing of the spinal anatomy. This can include a front view, a side view, and numerous cross-sectional views. The test was designed to show the anatomy of the bony structures of the spine and also allows us to see the discs and the nerves, although to a lesser extent than an MRI does. A doctor might prefer a CT scan over an MRI if a patient is very claustrophobic and cannot tolerate being in the MRI machine even with a sedative, or if there is a special need to identify with increased specificity the anatomy of the bony structures where the nerves exit the spinal canal. The latter of these two reasons would only pertain to a patient who is being considered for surgery.

Like the MRI the CT scanner is a cylindrical machine within which the patient lies on his or her back for a period of approximately thirty to forty-five minutes. Unlike the MRI the cylindrical portion of the machine is much larger and is much less likely to cause a claustrophobic sensation. The test is safe and painless. CT scans are sometimes done with "contrast agents" similar to the enhancement agents discussed under MRI.

As with MRI studies, similar caution is advised in regard to "abnormal" findings of CT scans, which may actually mean nothing unless correlated with the physical examination and history data.

Myelography

A myelogram is an X ray of the fluid-filled sac surrounding the spinal cord. In this test a liquid contrast agent, or dye, is injected into the sac by the radiologist. Since it is "radiopaque," it will show up on the X-ray picture as white.

A myelogram is frequently followed by a CT scan, done within one to two hours after introduction of the contrast agent and after obtaining an initial set of plain X rays. Done in this way, the test allows us to have "the best of all possible worlds" with respect to being able to image the skeletal structures (bones) as well as the neurologic structures, which have been outlined by the contrast agent.

This test is generally only appropriate as a presurgical screening test. It is useful in the elderly population who have spinal stenosis and when the physician wants to image the spine in a standing position with the patient bending forward and/or backward. It is also helpful in the rare instances in which an MRI or CT scan is equivocal and there is the question of the presence of a tumor. One of the misuses of this test, which is now becoming less frequent, is to use it simply as a diagnostic procedure in a person who would not be a candidate for surgical treatment. *Unless the person being referred for the myelogram would consent to undergo surgical treatment as a possible intervention, there is no point in undergoing this invasive test.*

In most situations there is minimal pain associated with the procedure. It begins with the patient lying on a table so that the dye can be injected into the spinal canal. This takes about a minute or two, and you may feel a slight prick as the needle is inserted. Once the dye is injected, the plain X rays are taken with the patient in many positions, including standing, partially upright, lying down, and turned to the right or left side. The CT scan may then be done. After the completion of the test (which takes about an hour), myelograms usually require a recovery period of six to twelve hours. You may be asked to lie with your head slightly elevated, and you'll need to drink plenty of fluids. This keeps the contrast material away from sensitive areas in the head and neck while flushing the material from your body.

Headache is one side effect that can occur due to a reaction to the dye or a spinal fluid leak. Headaches due to a reaction to the dye now occur with a frequency of less than 1 percent, ever since the newer water-soluble dyes have been introduced over the past five years. In the second situation up to 5 to 10 percent of patients undergoing the procedure may experience headache for one or two days following the test because some of the cerebral spinal fluid leaked out through the needle hole. This almost always subsides with a short period of rest and the intake of fluids.

Although this test does carry with it more risks than the ones we have previously discussed, it is still considered a very low-risk procedure. Specifically there are two very rare risks: they are infection, which can occur with any invasive procedure, and abnormal bleeding. To prevent bleeding, it is very important that the patient be off of aspirin or any blood thinners for a period of three to five days prior to the test.

In the past the test required hospitalization. Currently it is almost always completed on an outpatient basis. The only reason it might be done on an inpatient basis is if possible complications are expected to occur.

CT Discogram

A discogram is a test that requires that a dye be injected directly into the disc itself. This test can be moderately painful. The injection of dye into the disc(s) is done to image the spine using a CT scan as well as to ascertain whether or not the introduction of the dye causes the type of back pain the patient has been experiencing. Sometimes an anesthetic is injected after the dye (and the reproduction of the pain) in order to determine if it will then alleviate the pain.

The indications for this test are controversial. It is used primarily in patients who have shown disc bulges or herniations at more than one level on an MRI study. In this situation the discogram might be done in an attempt to identify which, if any, of the identified disc herniations are responsible for the patient's clinical pain problem. An example would be the patient with three lumbar-level herniated discs. In the discogram test all three discs would be injected, and if one of them reproduced the pain, then the doctor would assume this is the problem disc.

This test should be indicated rarely and only if one were willing to consider surgical intervention based upon the results of the test. Side effects of this test are primarily that of infection, which is very rare.

Bone Scan

A bone scan is a test that requires the injection of a radioisotope dye in the arm, followed by a period of lying down while the dye is allowed to circulate throughout the entire body, including the skeletal structures. This can take two hours or more. After the dye has had a chance to circulate, special X rays are taken to determine the radioactivity (safe, low levels) in various parts of the skeleton. The scan works by detecting an increased radioactivity in that area of the skeleton that has increased blood flow, due either to a tumor, an infection, or a fracture. It is generally used when these conditions cannot be diagnosed on plain X-ray films, MRI, or CT scan.

This test is reasonably inexpensive and safe. It is essentially risk-free, though some back-pain patients find it difficult to lie down for an extended period of time while the dye is circulating. As with the other tests, the results must be taken as part of the entire evaluation. The most common mistake is to attribute too much significance to a finding that is due to osteoarthritic or wear-and-tear changes in the facet joints.

Electrodiagnostic Studies

The most common electrodiagnostic studies in back pain include electromyography (EMG) and nerve conduction studies (NCS). This testing is utilized to measure the electrical activity and function of nerves and muscles. The tests can show if the electrical activity of various nerves has somehow been disrupted. They are useful in clarifying or reinforcing a diagnosis.

During the procedure the examining physician will insert small needles into several muscles being measured. In an EMG these needles are connected to a monitor that will show the electrical activity of the nerves and muscles. In the nerve conduction study the nerves being studied are "buzzed" with an electrical stimulus so that their electrical activity can be monitored by the receiving electrodes.

These tests are moderately painful but can be helpful in distinguishing a variety of diagnoses in which the nervous system might be compromised or to assess the "regrowth" of nerves after lumbar disc surgery for sciatica. For the most part electrodiagnostic testing has become less necessary, as the great majority of diagnoses in patients with back pain can be made by a good history and physical examination, in addition to other diagnostic tests available (e.g., MRI).

Psychological Testing

Are you surprised that we've included psychological testing with other diagnostic tests? No, it is not a mistake, nor has the section been placed incorrectly in this chapter.

A variety of psychological tests have been constructed or adapted for use with back-pain patients. These tests have been developed for many reasons including assessing such things as emotional aspects of the pain, concomitant psychiatric problems, ability to cope with the pain, and for use as presurgical screenings.

Just as the clinical history and physical examination is the most important part of diagnosing a back-pain program, the clinical interview is the key psychological assessment tool. A patient may be referred for a psychological assessment of his or her back pain for many reasons:

- Significant depression and/or anxiety

- Substance abuse including alcohol or overuse of pain medicines

- Inability to cope with the pain

- Stress in the family or work situation

- A need for psychological preparation for surgery

- A need to learn psychological pain-control procedures

- If stress-related back pain is suspected

Psychological assessment of a back-pain problem is usually conducted by a psychologist or psychiatrist with special training in pain problems. The clinical interview will usually involve getting information about the history of the pain problem including previous treatments, the family and work situations, litigation and compensation issues related to the back pain, history of previous psychological treatment, substance abuse problems, and history of emotional and/or physical abuse, among other things. In addition a mental-status examination is usually done, which assesses such things as mood, sleep, memory and concentration abilities, changes in sex drive and frequency, and energy levels.

Psychological testing might include a variety of things, and many tests are available for use. The evaluation and testing will give information on many aspects of a back-pain problem, including:

- Levels of depression and anxiety

- Personality features of the person with back pain

- Whether the person is more "comfortable" or "uncomfortable" in the sick role

- Whether the patient is more dramatic or stoic in showing pain behaviors

- How likely it is that the back pain is being influenced by nonphysical factors (emotions, family situation, work, etc.)

Many patients are very threatened when referred for this kind of assessment because they feel they are being "dumped" by their doctor. They also feel that the referral means that their doctor does not believe the pain is "real." As discussed throughout this book, the distinction between "real" and "imagined" pain is not a useful one. All pain is real and can be influenced by a variety of factors. Referral for psychological assessment of your back pain will generally be done for the reasons listed above. Usually the purpose of the evaluation is either to help the referring doctor better plan the treatment approach and/or to determine if psychological pain control methods might be helpful (e.g., relaxation training, changing ways you think about the pain, helping the family cope with you being in pain).

An example of psychological assessments for back pain can be found in chapter 15. You are more likely to be referred for this kind of evaluation if your back pain has gone on for quite some time. This is because the longer the pain goes on, the more likely psychological and emotional factors will come into play.

PART III

TREATMENT OF YOUR BACK PAIN

CHAPTER 8

COMMON TREATMENTS FOR BACK PAIN: USEFUL OR USELESS?

Leaders in back-pain research point out that the high number of different treatments for back pain suggests that diagnosing the cause of the pain in the majority of cases is not possible. It also brings into question just how successful all of these treatments are in relieving back pain and increasing functioning. The numerous treatments available have been categorized by the Quebec Task Force as follows:

- Promote rest

- Diminish spasm

- Diminish inflammation

- Reduce pain

- Increase strength

- Increase range of motion

- Increase endurance

- Alter joint tissue

- Alter nerve tissue

- Increase function

- Modify the work environment

- Modify the social environment

- Modify psychological and emotional issues

We took the liberty of borrowing part of the title of this chapter from Dr. Richard Deyo of the University of Washington, who wrote an article entitled "Conservative Therapy for Low Back Pain: Distinguishing Useful from Useless Therapy," published in the *Journal of the American Medical Association* in 1983. In that article Dr. Deyo makes the point that most research on conservative therapy for low back pain is wrought with problems, making it difficult to draw specific conclusions. Of course if medical professionals have difficulty drawing conclusions about specific treatments, it will be virtually impossible for the layperson to make informed choices about which treatments to pursue. This ambiguity increases the stress-related aspect of a back-pain experience, which can actually increase the pain due to the patient's emotional response to this ambiguity. This in turn tends to increase overall suffering.

In this chapter we will present the most commonly used conservative therapies for back pain. Under each treatment we will discuss a description of the procedure as well as its purpose and the purported effects. After that presentation we will discuss our orientation regarding the treatment, based not only on our clinical experience but also on the most recent available research literature. We will then provide guidelines to help you decide whether a specific treatment might be appropriate for you, as well as deciding how much of that treatment to pursue.

This chapter will not cover treatments of reconditioning, exercise, or medication use, as these are covered extensively in other chapters.

CONDUCTIVE HEAT

Description
Hot packs are commonly used as a means of symptom management in back and neck pain. Commercial hot packs used by physical therapists are generally designed to deliver moist heat to the affected areas. Moist heat is superficial heat, although it is capable of reaching farther under the skin by means of heat

conduction through the tissues. The effects of this heating process on the tissues include an increase in local metabolism, an increase in local vasodilation (expansion of the blood vessels), and promotion of muscle relaxation. If the hot packs are applied for an extended period of time, there may be an overall increase in body temperature, along with an increase in respiration and pulse rates as the body attempts to dissipate the excess heat caused by the application of the hot packs.

Purpose

The rationale behind this treatment is that the promotion of muscle relaxation, as well as increasing local blood flow, will help with pain relief. It is very commonly used in the treatment of both acute and chronic back and neck pain. Although the application of moist heat certainly can provide temporary pain relief, there is no scientific evidence of its long-term effectiveness. This procedure is probably one of the most overused treatments for back and neck pain in industrialized countries. Patients typically report that while the packs are applied, they do experience some relief of their pain, but as soon as they leave the clinic, the pain returns to its original levels after a short period of time.

Comment

We believe use of hot packs is reasonable on a very time-limited basis in acute back pain, as well as in helping the person to successfully engage in an aggressive exercise program. The key to utilizing hot packs is that they not be used for an extended period of time and should not be considered as any type of effective treatment for the pain. They are merely a *tool* in order to help the person engage in activities that have been shown to be effective for back pain

ULTRASOUND

Description

Ultrasound refers to sound waves that are of such high frequency that they are not detectable by the human ear. Sound waves are capable of reflection, penetration, and absorption. This means they may be reflected off of certain surfaces, they can penetrate certain substances, and they are absorbed by certain substances. As far as their use on humans, ultrasound waves are absorbed by various tissues in the body, which causes a production of heat at the tissue site. Compared with all of the other heat modalities, heating penetration below the surface of the skin is greatest using ultrasound. The greatest heating effect is seen in tissues such as muscles and nerves, with very little increase in temperature in fat tissue.

Purpose

The purposes of ultrasound are similar to those discussed above for moist heat. As ultrasound creates heat within the tissues, the effects are similar. Ultrasound can achieve these results at a much deeper level than moist heat for reasons discussed above. Generally it is believed that it takes three to six treatments before much improvement can be expected. Also the patient may feel an increase in symptoms following the initial treatment.

Comment

This is another modality that is very commonly used in the treatment of back and neck pain. The physician will often prescribe hot packs and ultrasound in an attempt to provide pain relief. Again there is virtually no well-controlled scientific evidence that this treatment provides any effective long-term resolution of a back-pain problem beyond what would happen naturally. Patients tell us that it does provide temporary relief, but again this relief is extremely short-lived. We may prescribe it on a time-limited basis and only in conjunction with a reconditioning program.

MASSAGE

Description

It is beyond the scope of this book to describe all the types of massage that are available to address back pain. Massage can be of various intensities (superficial or deep) and done in conjunction with other treatments (e.g., exercise).

Purpose

The rationale behind the use of massage to address the pain is similar to that of applying heat and ultrasound. Massage is thought to increase blood flow to the local area, as well as relaxing the muscles and therefore causing a decrease in spasm and pain. As with the previous two treatments there is virtually no well-controlled scientific evidence that massage produces a long-term reduction in back pain over what would occur normally through the healing process. Our patients tell us that the massage certainly feels good while it is being received and for a short time thereafter; but in the majority of cases the pain then returns to its pretreatment levels. Everyone, regardless of whether he or she has pain or not, finds a massage pleasurable, but that does not make it effective in the treatment of back pain.

Comment

Massage therapy is very commonly used as a treatment for both acute and chronic back pain. However, there have been virtually no scientifically acceptable investigations that support the use of massage as an actual treatment for back pain. In one study, patients suffering from nonspecific back pain were randomly assigned to one of four treatment groups: (1) treatment by their general physician that included a home exercise program; (2) a physiotherapy treatment group that included exercise, massage, and modalities; (3) a manual-therapy group consisting of spinal manipulation; and (4) a placebo treatment group. In the latter group the patients believed they were getting actual physical therapy treatment when in fact they were not. During the twelve weeks of follow-up after the initiation of treatments, all four groups showed similar significant improvement in terms of pain relief and return to normal functioning. Interestingly patients rated the physiotherapy, manual therapy, and placebo treatments as more effective than being monitored by the general physician. This underscores the powerful effect of expectations in treatments for back pain. This will be discussed further in the placebo section at the end of this chapter.

Given these research findings and our clinical observations, we will use massage on a very, very limited basis as a means to help patients begin to exercise and get reactivated. Certainly continued massage therapy on a long-term basis is not helpful in treating back pain. In fact it promotes unnecessary medical bills and reinforces the sick role of the patient.

"HUMMERS" AND "SHAKE AND BAKE"

The previous three treatments (hot packs, ultrasound, and massage) are referred to as "hummers" within professional groups who specialize in pain medicine. These treatments are also often referred to as "shake and bake" treatments because they are applied almost as a knee-jerk response by physicians who want to try something for the pain but are unsure of which approach to take. Treatment approaches are complicated by the fact that most back pain is of unknown etiology. Therefore these treatments focus on attempting to provide relief without regard to diagnosis. These "shake and bake" treatments are overprescribed and overutilized, which causes an extreme financial burden on the patient as well as a feeling of hopelessness when they do not work.

One might ask, "If these treatments have not been shown to be effective, why are they so common?" This phenomenon has to do with what people *think* is effective versus what actually *is* effective. Since the treatments feel good while they are being applied and back pain naturally gets better on its own (in 90 percent of cases), people falsely attribute the "cure" to the treatment rather than to the natural healing process. In most cases, the pain would have improved even without these treatments.

Comment
In our clinical experience patients will often come in saying they have had a course of hot packs, ultrasound, and massage

treatment, which felt good while the treatment was being applied but generally did not provide lasting relief. We have heard of patients who have undergone this type of treatment for a few months and of one woman who had been receiving these treatments on a twice-per-week basis for fifteen years. Not surprisingly her back pain was essentially unchanged since the beginning of treatment. She and her physician rationalized the approach by stating, "It appears the pain is going to be chronic, so we might as well give her some temporary relief, as that is all that can be expected."

We do believe that these treatments may have their place in back pain even though their long-term effectiveness is dubious. We will use them on a very time-limited basis and almost always in conjunction with helping the patient through a treatment program that has been shown to be effective. This might include the application of these "modalities" prior to engaging in a therapeutic exercise program. The maximum time for this type of treatment would be extremely limited. Also we quickly move to having patients use modalities (heat, ice, etc.) on their own without it continuing to be part of the "formal" treatment.

CRYOTHERAPY

Description
Cryotherapy is a fancy name for several methods of delivering cold treatments for therapeutic purposes. This is generally done through the use of ice packs, although it can also be done through other methods. Cryotherapy can be delivered in a number of ways, including ice packs, commercial cold packs, iced towels, ice massage, cold baths, and vapocoolant spray.

Purpose
The effect of the application of cold includes local vasoconstriction (decreased blood flow) with a subsequent vasodilation. It seems paradoxical that vasodilation occurs with the application of cold just as it does with the application of heat.

This is because the application of cold causes an initial decrease in blood flow with a reflexive increase in blood flow after a short period of time. Patients will also experience a predictable set of sensations, including cold, burning, aching, and numbness in the local area.

Vapocoolant spray includes such substances as ethyl chloride or fluoromethane liquids, which when sprayed on the skin produce significant cooling through evaporation. Generally the physical therapist will spray the substance along a local area from a bottle that produces a fine stream of the liquid. Vapocoolant sprays are generally used in what is called a spray-and-stretch procedure. This includes spraying the substance along the affected area and then having the patient do a passive stretch of the muscles. It is generally used for patients who present with a limitation in their range of motion, as well as trigger points.

Comment

Applying ice to the area of back pain can be useful in the early stages of treatment to help with pain relief and prevent swelling. It is not a long-term treatment in and of itself, but can allow actual treatment (e.g., back exercises) to progress more smoothly. It is generally recommended that ice be applied early on, followed by heat after the first few days postinjury, although some doctors recommend applying heat or ice depending on what feels better to the patient. Again, these are used on a time-limited basis.

BED REST

Description

At first any description of bed rest would seem to be obvious: Get in bed and rest. It is not exactly as straightforward as it might seem, and we will discuss this in the following section. As we presented in the chapter on medical myths, bed rest is the most frequently used treatment for low back pain. We have found that prescriptions for bed rest given to patients are generally vague, but will often be for two to three weeks along with the admonition to "let pain be your guide."

Purpose
There are various rationales behind prescribing bed rest, the two most common of which include:

• Many patients appear to report pain relief with bed rest.

• Studies have shown that pressure on the disc between the vertebrae is decreased in the supine (lying on your back) position. It appears, then, that bed rest is primarily prescribed to rest an injured part of the body.

Comment
The foregoing reasoning behind bed rest is flawed for two reasons. First, as we have discussed, the vast majority of back-pain cases are of unknown etiology, and no structural damage is noted. Second, letting pain be your guide is only applicable in the very early stages of back pain due to factors discussed in chapter 4.

Dr. Alf Nachemson has reviewed the level of proof of effectiveness of various common treatment modalities for low back pain of an unspecified period. It has been found by more than one study that for back pain of less than six weeks a maximum of less than two days' bed rest is optimal. There is no proof that bed rest beyond two days is effective, and in fact it has been found that there are various adverse consequences to longer periods of bed rest with longer periods of pain. As we discussed previously, these include the perception by the patient and others that he or she is suffering from a severe illness, economic loss, muscle deterioration and atrophy, physical deconditioning, and bone mineral loss. Although bed rest may be appropriate on a very time-limited basis (two days), longer-term bed rest can have disastrous consequences.

It is important to be specific in how the bed rest is prescribed. If you are lying on your back and simply turn to your side, you have put pressure on your disc that is 75 percent of the normal pressure on your disc when you are standing! Also people will often not follow the bed-rest prescription faithfully. As we have seen for a variety of these treatments, bed-rest prescriptions are often based on flawed information and reasoning as to the cause of the back pain. In addition, although some of the treatments may be useful when used in a limited manner, the reasoning that "if a little is good, then a lot must be great" is absolutely wrong.

TRACTION

Description
Cervical traction is used to address neck pain, while pelvic traction is used to address lower back pain. Traction is a procedure by which pressure is applied to the spine in order to pull the vertebrae away from each other. Traction can be done manually by the therapist or with the use of an apparatus. In mechanical cervical traction a halter is placed on the patient's head, which is attached to a machine by a rope that pulls on the halter. Pelvic traction is achieved in a similar manner, although pressure is applied via a corset around the hips. Home units are available for applying traction.

Purpose
The purpose of cervical traction is generally to relieve pain. The rationale behind this approach is that the pulling on the neck allows for the following:

- It gives rest to the area by supporting the weight of the body region

- It puts the spine in a good postural alignment

- It improves blood flow to the muscles around the neck area

- It decreases the pressure on the discs between the vertebrae

Comment

There have been several studies of traction. Dr. Deyo (1991) reports that "At least seven randomized clinical trials of conventional traction have been published with striking consistency in their results" (page 1573). In these studies patients were assigned to either a condition of traction treatment or another condition in which a fake traction procedure was done. In the latter of these conditions patients believed they were receiving traction although no actual traction was being done. *Consistent results showed that none of these studies demonstrated any significant benefit for traction over the fake treatment.* Dr. Deyo concluded that "These data clearly support the consensus view of the Quebec Task Force On Spinal Disorders which concluded that there was no scientific evidence to support the use of spinal traction despite its wide spread application in practice."

Again we see hundreds of patients who have previously been treated with many sessions of traction only to report that they received "temporary relief."

HYDROTHERAPY

Description

Hydrotherapy means simply "water therapy." Water is commonly used as a therapeutic medium in one of two ways. These include either whirlpool, exercising in water, or both.

Purpose

The rationale behind using water for treatment is related to its physical properties. One of the properties of water is buoyancy, which helps to support the weight of the patient while submerged. Due to this buoyancy, as well as to other factors, a person is essentially weightless when in water. Another property of water is called viscosity. This can be thought of in simple terms as a resistance to movement. Viscosity causes a resistance to movement through water and this resistance increases as one tries to move faster. You have undoubtedly experienced the effects of both buoyancy and viscosity if you have ever played or swum in a swimming pool.

A whirlpool is simply a water bath in which the water is moved and agitated by a turbine. The water is most commonly heated, causing it to be a source of moist heat. Generally the effects of whirlpool treatment are similar to those discussed above for heat.

The other aspect of treatment using water includes doing various exercises while in water. This may include such things as an exercise class in a shallow pool, as well as more high-tech approaches, such as underwater treadmills. The rationale behind this type of treatment is that exercises can be done in a safer and more fluid manner due to the viscosity of the water. In addition the buoyancy allows for exercises to be done with virtually no weight being placed on the spine.

Comment

In the early stages of back pain the patient may benefit from beginning an exercise program in water. This should be viewed as a stepping-stone to getting to the point where the exercise can be done outside the pool or water tank. Exercising in water, including swimming, is an excellent source of conditioning.

TRANSCUTANEOUS ELECTRICAL NERVE STIMULATION

Description

Transcutaneous electrical nerve stimulation (TENS) is a procedure that includes the application of low levels of electricity to the areas of pain. Generally electrodes are placed on the skin and a small generator unit causes a low level of electricity to be passed between the electrodes. The patient will often experience a tingling or prickling sensation. There are currently a wide variety of TENS units on the market, which emit electrical patterns of differing amplitudes, frequencies, and pulse widths.

Purpose

The rationale behind TENS is based on the gate-control theory, as discussed in chapter 4. It is thought that the electrical stimulation causes the nervous system to block pain impulses from reaching the brain, therefore decreasing pain perception. TENS units are generally very small and portable and can be worn throughout the day for pain relief. It should be emphasized that the TENS procedure is strictly for the reduction of pain and does not treat the origin of the pain.

Comment

There have been many studies of TENS with conflicting results. In prescribing TENS we will generally gauge the effectiveness on an individual basis. As these units tend to be very expensive, renting one for a brief period to gauge its effectiveness is a most prudent course. We see many patients who have purchased a TENS unit, used it for a brief period, then retired it to the junk drawer.

The TENS treatment should be provided in conjunction with other treatments that will actually help increase functioning and are effective over the long term.

CORSETS AND BRACES

Description

Corsets and braces are very widely used for both back and neck pain. When used in neck pain they are referred to as cervical collars.

Purpose

A brace is generally used for the lower back for the purpose of restricting motion, providing abdominal support, and correcting posture. A neck brace is worn to restrict movement as well as relieving the neck of the weight of the head.

Comment

Except in very specific disorders there is very little scientific evidence to support the effectiveness of braces or corsets.

There is a rationale for using corsets and rigid braces after spinal surgery, as well as in such disorders as spondylolisthesis (see chapter 6). Using a corset or brace in back pain of unknown etiology can exacerbate the disuse syndrome, which includes atrophy of important muscles that normally support the back. Using a brace also restricts motion that over the long term can cause muscle shortening and thereby cause further problems aside from the original pain.

MANIPULATION

Description
It is beyond the scope of this book to describe all the different types of spinal manipulation currently being practiced. Manipulation (or "manual medicine") is defined as procedures where the hands are used to mobilize, adjust, apply traction, massage, stimulate, or otherwise influence the spine and surrounding tissues to promote healing and pain relief. Spinal manipulation is generally practiced by chiropractors, osteopaths, and, less frequently, physical therapists.

The chiropractic treatment of back pain is extremely common. Estimates are that 30 percent of the low-back-pain population in the United States is seen by chiropractors. In addition approximately 50 percent of visits to chiropractors are for low back pain.

Purpose
Spinal manipulation is highly controversial among traditional medical practitioners because it is equated with the practice of chiropractic (Deyo, 1983). Dr. Deyo discusses the fact that there is no clear biological rationale for the use of manipulation, although possible suggested benefits include the following:

- Reduction of a bulging disc between the vertebrae by tightening certain ligaments

- Loosening certain tissues around a disc

- Stimulation of certain nerve fibers that might inhibit pain impulses

Spinal manipulation is used to treat virtually every type of back-pain problem. Even so there are risks associated with the procedure. These are quite rare and include injury to cerebral (a structure in the brain) blood flow following manipulation of the neck, and development of a cauda equina syndrome as the result of lumbar manipulation.

Comment

It is difficult to judge the effectiveness of spinal manipulation, as well-controlled scientific studies are lacking. Certainly, as discussed above, there are millions of people who go to their chiropractor on a regular basis and attest to the effectiveness of this approach. The problem is determining whether the treatment effect is actually due to the spinal manipulation or simply to the expectation in the patient that it will work (placebo response).

Scientific studies seem to be showing that patients who receive spinal manipulation can gain faster, short-term relief of symptoms compared with patients who did not receive the manipulation. In these studies the differences in symptom relief disappeared at three weeks, at which time both groups were the same. Dr. Deyo has concluded that "There is accumulating evidence that some types of spinal manipulation may have short-term, but not long-term benefits."

Based on our experience in dealing with a great many patients who have had or are currently receiving chiropractic treatment, we recommend that it be done on a short-term, time-limited basis, usually for acute back pain of less than two to four months' duration. We encourage patients not to become dependent on the treatment and we emphasize moving quickly from treatment to an independent type of exercise program.

There are contraindications ("not recommended") for spinal manipulation, for which patients should be screened. These generally include unstable fractures, severe osteoporosis, osteomyelitis, bone tumors, any progressive neurologic deficit, certain types of disc herniations, hypermobile joints, rheumatoid arthritis, and certain bleeding disorders. You should receive a comprehensive physical and spinal examination prior to beginning such treatment and keep the treatment time-limited.

ACUPUNCTURE

Description
Acupuncture is the process of placing needles in various parts of the body to affect the patient's perception of pain as well as to cure a wide variety of other problems. It has its roots in ancient Chinese culture dating back thousands of years. The technique for stimulation might include movement of the needles, electrical stimulation of the needles, or application of pressure (acupressure).

Purpose
Acupuncture is sometimes used for the treatment of back pain. Most of the research on the benefits of acupuncture for back pain has involved chronic cases. These studies randomly assign patients to either an acupuncture treatment group or a placebo group. Results of these studies are quite consistent in showing advantages when compared with physical therapies or with "fake" treatments that the patients believe are effective (placebo). However, when actual acupuncture using placement of needles according to Chinese meridians is compared with acupuncture in which the needles are purposely put in the wrong place, the treatment groups show no differences.

One theory on the mechanism of action in acupuncture is that it is related to the gate-control theory and to endorphins (morphinelike chemicals that are naturally produced in the body). It is thought that the acupuncture helps block the pain impulse from getting to the brain as well as promoting the release of endorphins.

Comment

We see many patients who have tried acupuncture for back-pain relief. Consistent with the above research, it appears to be helpful for some people while not for others. It appears that much of the response can be attributed to placebo factors.

If you are interested in attempting acupuncture for your back pain, it is recommended that you keep the treatment brief and do it in conjunction with a reactivation exercise program, as discussed in this book. If you have chronic back pain, it will be essential to address all aspects of the problem, not just the pain.

BIOFEEDBACK

Description

Biofeedback is the process of using monitoring machines (often a computer) to retrain physical states in your body that are not normally under voluntary control. For instance biofeedback has been used to train people to do such things as lower their heart rate, decrease muscle tension, and lower blood pressure.

Biofeedback training for muscle problems involves placing electrodes on the skin over the area of muscle to be retrained. This might be an area of soreness or spasm. The computer can then measure the amount of muscle electrical activity that is present. This electrical activity is related to the tension in the muscle. The patient can see the amount of tension on the monitor and begin to learn to decrease it. It is a painless, noninvasive procedure, as the sensors are taped to the skin and only monitor activity.

Purpose

On the assumption that back pain often involves "muscle spasm," biofeedback treatment theoretically makes sense in terms of learning how to reduce the tension. It is assumed that a decrease in pain accompanies the decrease in muscle spasm.

There are very few well-controlled scientific studies on the effectiveness of biofeedback in back-pain problems even though it is widely used. Clinically, positive results are often seen, but it is not clear whether this is due to actual treatment effects of decreased muscle tension, giving the patient a sense of increased control over the pain, or to the placebo response. Another difficult result to explain is that subjective treatment effects (e.g., the patient saying the tension and pain are less) often occur even when the training has not resulted in an actual change in tension levels as measured by the computer.

Until further evidence is available, we will sometimes recommend a short trial of biofeedback (four to eight sessions) if muscle tension appears to be part of the back-pain problem or if the patient is showing anxiety about the symptoms. The essential feature of biofeedback training is the rapid teaching of the patient to relax without needing the equipment. This is done through relaxation training and the use of audiotapes.

Biofeedback is abused by practitioners who give too many sessions and keep the patient dependent on the biofeedback machines. Some research has even indicated that the biofeedback machine itself may not be necessary and that the same result can be achieved through relaxation training. Even so we find a powerful effect for the patient in being able to see the changes occur as learning takes place.

Patients occasionally have trouble making the transition from traditional medical treatments to that of biofeedback and relaxation training. This is because in the former treatments something is done to the patient, whereas in the latter the patient must learn the skill. This requires motivation and commitment to practice. If the patient is unwilling to do this, the treatment will not be effective.

TRIGGER-POINT INJECTIONS

Description
Trigger-point injections involve the injection of a small amount of anesthetic into "trigger points." These are areas of muscle that seem to "trigger" pain throughout a region of the body.

Often a patient will be able to point to a specific localized area that when touched causes significant radiating pain.

Purpose

The purpose of the trigger-point injections is to break up the "pain cycle" usually associated with myofascial pain disorders. It is thought that these areas cause localized and/or referred pain.

Comment

We use trigger-point injections on a time-limited basis and usually only in association with an overall rehabilitation program. This type of treatment is also sometimes abused in the treatment of back pain where patients undergo multiple injections on a regular basis for a very extended period of time. There is no scientific evidence that this approach is beneficial. Trigger-point injections may help in the initial stages of exercise rehabilitation, similar to that of other modalities.

EPIDURAL STEROID INJECTIONS

Description

Epidural steroid injections involve the injection of steroid compounds (often combined with a local anesthetic) into the epidural space (an area in the spinal canal), generally done to treat nerve-root irritation. The technique includes using a small spinal needle to inject the steroid into the intraspinal area. Although most patients are concerned about the prospect of having an injection "in their spine," most of them report that it was a relatively easy procedure to undergo. The epidural injections are often done in a series of up to three, separated by a specific number of days or weeks. The decision to have more than one injection is generally guided by the patient's response to the first one. Recent research and clinical evidence also suggest that the full benefit of the epidural steroid injection may not occur for as long as seven to ten days afterward.

Purpose

The rationale is that local inflammation is an important factor in pain complaints of sciatica and back pain and that the steroids help in terms of decreasing the inflammation and pain.

Comment

Although the efficacy of epidural injections has not yet been firmly established in scientific studies, positive benefits often include decreased inflammation and a more rapid benefit in terms of decreased symptoms as compared with other techniques (local anesthetic or bed rest). Other issues that need to be addressed in the research include how many epidural steroid injections should be given and how to determine whether there was benefit or not. Most clinicians and researchers agree that there is some positive benefit found in most studies. The primary benefit of obtaining an epidural injection might be that it shortens disability from sciatica and back pain while having minimal risks.

We believe that the decision to obtain an epidural steroid injection should be guided by good clinical reasoning and necessity rather than the "give it a try" attitude. You should obtain a full explanation from your spine doctor of the reasons you are being referred for such a procedure. As with many of these treatments the use of epidural steroid injections should be done in conjunction with an overall rehabilitation approach. All too often the physician will attempt various techniques sequentially without an overall "master plan." In addition you should question the physician who continues to give you epidural nerve blocks either in the face of lack of improvement or beyond a series of three within a six-month period.

FACET INJECTIONS

Description

The idea that facet joints could be a source of back pain goes back to the 1930s. As we discussed in chapter 6, the concept of a "facet syndrome" as a source of back pain is still controversial. Facet injections are generally done on an outpatient basis in a radiology suite. They are done using a fluoroscopy table, which allows the doctor to place the injection precisely into the facet joint. After the procedure patients are generally encouraged to be physically active, but are also informed that the benefit of the injection will be unknown for at least one week.

Purpose
Based on the rationale that back pain could originate from the facet joints, it is proposed that injection of steroids and/or a local anesthetic into this area can provide pain relief.

Comment
Overall, studies have generally not shown good results from facet-joint injections. It appears that the best role for this type of therapy may be to provide a relatively brief period of relief from motion-limiting pain in order to allow the patient to proceed with an appropriate exercise program. Most studies find long-term benefit in less than 20 percent of patients undergoing the procedure. The short-term success rate is approximately 50 percent. One must weigh the benefits and risks associated with such a procedure versus conservative noninvasive approaches as discussed elsewhere in this book.

PAIN PROGRAMS, FUNCTIONAL RESTORATION, AND WORK HARDENING

Description
There is much confusion surrounding the difference between pain programs, functional-restoration treatment, and work hardening. There has been a great abuse of these terms in health care, and we will attempt to provide a simple description of each.

Although there is no official body that oversees the operation of pain programs, the International Association of the Study of

Pain has attempted to establish "desirable characteristics" for pain-treatment facilities. In doing so they have defined treatment centers in a specific manner. A *multidisciplinary pain center* is the most complex of facilities and would almost always be associated with a medical school or teaching hospital. It is an organization of different health care professionals and includes activities of patient care, research, and teaching components. It is most often based in a hospital. A *multidisciplinary pain clinic* is similar but does not include the teaching and research components. A *pain clinic* usually specializes in a specific diagnosis only ("the back-pain center," "the headache center," etc.). A *modality-oriented clinic* will focus on one specific type of treatment, such as a nerve-block clinic, acupuncture center, or biofeedback center. Many centers call themselves multidisciplinary pain programs when in fact they are not.

A *functional-restoration program* has as its primary purpose the elimination of disability and the restoration of function. A functional-restoration program seeks to quantify the patient's physical capacity and psychosocial function and then reactivate and recondition the patient toward resumption of normal work and social activities. These programs focus primarily on what the patient can do functionally rather than on pain relief. The philosophy is that pain reduction will follow improved functioning. It is guided by the assessment that "hurt does not equal harm" in chronic back-pain syndromes.

Work hardening is the supervised simulation of work activities, which are increased throughout the program in a graduated fashion. The patient may start out at the work-hardening clinic on a two-hour-per-day basis doing activities that approximate his or her actual job and then increase to an eight-hour workday (or his or her maximum tolerance). At that time the patient is transferred back to work.

As may be surmised, there can be a great deal of overlap among the aforementioned programs.

Purpose

The general purposes of each of these treatment approaches have been presented above. It is important to note that in most comprehensive multidisciplinary pain programs, functional-restoration treatments, and work-hardening programs, pain reduction is a secondary goal. The primary goal is to reverse the physical and mental deconditioning syndromes and to help the patient "function regardless of the pain." In doing this, pain reduction is also achieved.

Comment

As with any type of treatment, there can be a high degree of variability in the quality of these types of programs. There are several factors that can impact outcome, which include the quality of the program, the motivation of the patient, and the criteria used by the program to select participants. We have seen great success in chronic-back-pain-syndrome and failed-back-surgery-syndrome patients who are carefully selected for treatment and are motivated to complete these types of programs. Warning signs that you are dealing with a lower quality program are that virtually all patients who are referred get taken, the program focuses primarily on pain reduction rather than on functional goals, or that it does not provide multidisciplinary treatment in a coordinated fashion.

The overall research on multidisciplinary pain programs (which often include functional-restoration and work-hardening approaches) generally shows positive benefits. The overall average of pain reduction is about 30 percent with a 200 to 500 percent increase in physical functioning. Reduction in pain medicine is also addressed in treatment. Results generally show that 49 to 65 percent of treated patients remain medication-free by the one-year follow-up. Return to work is also a common goal of the treatment program if the patient has been disabled from work due to pain. Results generally show an average return-to-work rate of 55 percent in patients who, as a group, have been disabled for many years.

NATURAL HEALING AND THE PLACEBO RESPONSE

Natural healing is a key factor to take into account when discussing treatments for back pain.

> **In assessing the power of various treatments it must be kept in mind that about 70 percent of acute back-pain cases will resolve within three weeks and 90 percent within eight weeks even if no treatment is done at all!**

Therefore any treatment will need to demonstrate that it is more effective than the natural course of healing by speeding up the process or keeping the patient more comfortable while the healing is taking place.

The placebo response has to do with a patient's expectation or belief that a treatment is effective whether or not it really is. Placebo responses usually account for about 30 to 40 percent of the success response to a purported treatment. Therefore if a doctor told you that standing on your head daily for two weeks would be beneficial for your back pain, and you believed in the prescription, it most likely would work (at least to some degree). This demonstrates the power of the mind in treatments for back pain. It also explains why there are so many treatments for back pain, all of which seem to be somewhat effective. The likelihood of a placebo response can be heightened depending upon how the treatment is presented by the practitioner. For instance it is more likely if the doctor says, "I know what is wrong and this is the way we fix it."

SUMMARY AND CONCLUSIONS

As we have seen, there are a variety of conservative treatments for back pain. The key thing to remember is that 90 percent of acute, nonspecific back pain resolves within two months whether or not formal treatment is completed. In most cases in which back pain goes on longer than two months, a primary element of the treatment will be an appropriate exercise program and limited use of certain medicines. In a percentage of cases other treatments may be necessary. The appropriate use of these treatments is discussed in other chapters. It should be kept in mind that the longer the pain continues, the more likely there are to be a myriad of factors impacting the pain. These include other physical problems (e.g., deconditioning) and psychological issues (depression, fear, anxiety, etc.). This type of chronic back pain often requires a coordinated, multi-disciplinary intervention.

CHAPTER 9

AGGRESSIVE
CONSERVATIVE
TREATMENT

This chapter summarizes what we believe to be the core element in the treatment of back problems and successful recovery. Physical and mental deconditioning appear to be critical elements in back pain of a subacute or chronic nature. Thus physical and mental *reconditioning* are essential for overcoming these problems. The key element in terms of utilizing this approach will be managing your fear of the pain, accepting the fact that hurt does not equal harm, and openly addressing issues that may be pressuring you to maintain the sick role. All of these influences are discussed throughout this book. Putting this information into practice will help you overcome your back pain regardless of whether it is acute, subacute, chronic, or recurrent acute. The key variable in the equation is you.

Aggressive conservative treatment should generally be preceded by a careful physical evaluation by the physician. This is done primarily to rule out any underlying serious condition that may be responsible for your back pain. These types of rare serious conditions are discussed in chapters 6 and 12. This initial evaluation is usually done with a good history and physical examination, and does not often require the need for any further diagnostic testing. Certainly, however, the individual physician must determine the role, if any, for any specific diagnostic test.

Once it is determined by the physician that the back pain is not due to an emergent condition requiring other treatment, an aggressive conservative treatment plan is most often indicated. This treatment approach may or may not be indicated for stress-related back pain depending on the degree of physical deconditioning that has occurred due to inactivity. This issue is further discussed below as well as in the last section of the book.

An aggressive conservative treatment program for back pain will generally be designed by the supervising physician (family doctor or specialist), osteopath, or chiropractor after the aforementioned issues have been addressed. It is most often implemented by a qualified physical therapist or exercise physiologist, although in many cases patients can simply be given a program of exercises and complete them on their own, independent of a formal treatment setting. This approach is most often attempted at the early stages of treatment and can often be guided by the family doctor.

There are several important aspects that must be attended to during the course of such a program. These include the following:

1. After you have been evaluated by your physician and such a program has been recommended, it is important to understand that you have an excellent prognosis for full recovery.

2. You must accept the fact that you may experience a mild to moderate increase in pain upon initiation of such a program. This pain does not indicate tissue damage and is what we would expect as part of increasing activity.

3. It is important to your treatment that you comply with your exercise program. This is probably the area of most concern, as people generally have trouble following through on exercise recommendations.

4. During the course of aggressive reconditioning, pay attention to emotional or other factors that may act as blockades to recovery. If these problems are occurring and are not addressed, the physical reconditioning will not work.

As we have discussed in previous chapters, there are various phases of back pain. These include acute (less than six weeks' duration), subacute (six to twelve weeks), and chronic (three to six months or more). Recurrent acute back pain is also common, and this is characterized by episodes of back pain that ultimately resolve and then recur at some future date.

The aggressive conservative treatment approach will change somewhat, depending on the phase of back pain you are experiencing. In the following pages we will briefly describe the treatment approaches for each of these phases of back pain. However, first we will discuss the physical-deconditioning syndrome or "disuse syndrome," which is key to understanding the rationale behind these treatment approaches.

THE DECONDITIONING SYNDROME

As far as we can determine, the deconditioning or disuse syndrome was first characterized in 1984. Since that time it has received much attention in relation to back-pain problems as well as other illnesses. It has been generalized beyond back-pain problems, and some feel it is related to "the base of much human ill-being."

The disuse syndrome is caused by physical inactivity and is fostered by our sedentary society. This disuse of our bodies leads to a deterioration of many body functions. This is basically an extension of the old adage "Use it or lose it." There are several physical consequences from disuse and deconditioning. These occur in many body systems, most notably those of the muscles and skeleton, cardiovascular, blood components, the gastrointestinal system, the endocrine systems, and the nervous system. For instance, in the musculoskeletal system disuse of muscles can rapidly lead to atrophy and muscle wasting. If you have ever had an arm or a leg in a cast, you will be familiar with the fact that the diameter of the affected limb may be noticeably smaller after being immobilized for some time.

Cardiovascular effects also occur due to disuse, including a decrease in oxygen uptake, a rise in systolic blood pressure, and an overall blood plasma volume decrease of 10 to 15 percent with extended bed rest. Physical inactivity also leads to nervous system changes, including slower mental processing, problems with memory and concentration, depression, and anxiety. Many other detrimental physiological changes also occur that are beyond the scope of this discussion. Disuse has been summarized as follows: "Inactivity plays a pervasive role in our lack of wellness. Disuse is physically, mentally, and spiritually debilitating." We strongly agree with this determination.

> **We feel that the deconditioning/disuse syndrome is a key variable in the perpetuation of most chronic back-pain problems.**

In summary the disuse or deconditioning syndrome associated with back pain can result in a myriad of significant medical problems and increase the likelihood of a chronic pain syndrome developing. As we have discussed throughout the book, common attitudes and treatments in the medical community reinforce the fear patients have about their back pain and the chance of reinjury, thus leading to passive treatment and deconditioning.

There are other problems associated with the deconditioning syndrome. For example, as we have discussed elsewhere in the book, tissue that is completely immobilized during the course of healing has a tendency to produce a scar that has low strength and resilience. This may be a factor in recurrent pain. On the other hand tissue that heals during the course of appropriate continued movement will have greater strength and flexibility. In addition a study by Dr. Tom Mayer has illustrated the specific negative effects of disuse on spinal muscles. It was found that significant deficiencies in the strength of back muscles occurred with disuse after a relatively short period of time.

The disuse syndrome and deconditioning syndrome can also lead to a variety of emotional changes that are associated with an increased perception of pain. As mentioned earlier, Dr. Robert Gatchel has termed this syndrome the mental-deconditioning syndrome, characterized by initial psychological distress, worry, and anxiety. Over time the syndrome results in depression, anger, substance abuse, and ultimate acceptance of the sick role.

The most ideal approach to managing the physical- and mental-deconditioning syndromes is to prevent their occurrence altogether. But even if the disuse syndrome has developed, the reconditioning approach is very effective. This will be discussed in the following sections.

PHYSICAL RECONDITIONING

Acute Back Pain

In the initial stages of acute back pain (generally less than six weeks), limited bed rest may be appropriate. As we have said, research indicates that two or three days is optimal unless there are other symptoms, such as pain radiating down the legs. In these cases more extended bed rest may be appropriate, but rarely more than four to six days.

At this stage of back pain, techniques that help with pain relief may also be useful. This might include such things as hot or cold packs. During this phase of treatment, pain medications, anti-inflammatories, and muscle relaxants may also be used. The use of the pain medications and muscle relaxants should be time-limited (this is discussed further in chapter 11).

Even during this early stage of back pain it is appropriate to walk and in many cases get mild exercise!

This continued movement will help prevent the development of deconditioning of your muscles. In addition, except in rare cases, movement of this type will not result in any injury.

After two weeks it is usually beneficial to increase the amount of exercise. At this point it is usually appropriate to add aerobic conditioning exercise, which might include such activities as bicycling, swimming, and speed walking. Many experts feel that the choice of exercise is actually not as important as being sure that it provides an aerobic conditioning component. The only caution is that you avoid moderate to severe twisting and bending during the course of these exercises at this early stage of recovery. Strengthening and proper body mechanics are also important in this phase.

Subacute Back Pain
The subacute back-pain phase is generally defined as six to twelve weeks after pain onset.

> **This is a critical stage of treatment, as this group is at a higher risk for development of a chronic pain syndrome.**

This is the stage during which it is determined whether you go on to recovery or develop a more chronic condition. At this stage referral to a more formal treatment program may be most appropriate. In the acute-pain stage treatment can generally be guided by the family physician or other nonspecialist. If the back pain has not resolved by six weeks, then a more specialized program may be indicated. The various types of exercises for back problems will be discussed later. They generally include aerobic, stretching, and strengthening components.

There are no clear guidelines as to medication usage at this stage of treatment. Medication decisions should be made between you and your doctor, with you playing an active role. Different doctors have varying levels of competence in prescribing medications for back pain during the subacute and chronic stages. Generally, taking a serious look at the actual need for muscle relaxants and continued pain medications is most appropriate. In our experience these medicines are often prescribed inappropriately and can actually make the problem worse.

Chronic Back Pain
The chronic-back-pain stage is generally defined as more than three to six months of back pain or past the point of expected healing time for the particular injury. At this stage it is critical for you to become very active in addressing your back-pain problem if you have not already done so.

The guidelines for approaching a chronic-back-pain problem have been nicely summarized by Dr. Richard Deyo and Dr. Stanley Bigos (and are part of the new AHCPR national guidelines). Their recommendations and guidelines for treatment of back pain at this stage will be outlined here.

One key point should be kept in mind at this stage:

The fact that the back pain has persisted for this length of time is not, in and of itself, a reason to pursue spine surgery.

This is often used as a rationale for attempting spine surgery by overzealous surgeons, especially when there is some finding on the imaging studies. However, in the vast majority of cases an aggressive conservative approach continues to be the most appropriate.

At this stage of back pain the aggressive reconditioning approach is most critical. By this time if you have not been exercising, the physical and mental deconditioning syndromes are probably fully established. Therefore you may be suffering from several of the effects listed above as part of the deconditioning syndromes. Overall this will have the impact of making your pain perception worse. In addition there will likely not be physical findings that can explain your level of pain or disability.

Fully participating in a reconditioning program, which includes strengthening, stretching, and aerobic exercise, is essential. These programs may cause an initial increase in your pain, and that is to be expected. Also, passive modality-oriented therapies such as hot packs, massage, and ultrasound are not indicated at this stage of pain. Use of ice or self-administered hot packs to help relieve symptomatic pain in conjunction with aggressive exercise may be appropriate.

It is essential at this stage of pain to investigate whether there are other factors that are exacerbating your pain or preventing recovery. This would include emotional problems, financial stress, job dissatisfaction, family stress, and assumption of the sick role. These pressures can have a significant impact on your back pain and, if not attended to, will certainly prevent recovery.

Exercises at this stage of treatment will also be done in a slightly different way. In the very early stages of back pain, allowing your amount and type of exercises to be guided by your pain is probably most appropriate. In the later stages of back pain this is usually exactly the wrong thing to do, although it continues to be prescribed by many doctors and physical therapists. In the chronic stages you must move from the philosophy of being guided by the pain to working and exercising regardless of the pain. During the chronic stage you must keep in mind that:

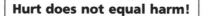

Hurt does not equal harm!

It is most appropriate to exercise and recondition yourself using what has been termed the quota system. This involves setting up an exercise regimen that progressively becomes more and more strenuous according to a fixed pattern. For instance you might start walking one-half block each day and then increase this by one block each week. With the quota system you would complete these exercises according to the plan whether or not your pain was better or worse. In this approach the pain is essentially taken out of the equation, since the exercises are designed to be safe for your back. Therefore it is known that no damage is being done even if the pain increases somewhat initially. The quota-system approach has been shown to be very effective in university pain-program settings. Unfortunately it is used much less in routine physical-therapy practice. The quota system will be discussed in more detail in a later section.

Pain medication should be tapered to the lowest possible level during this stage of pain and treatment. In addition medications should be prescribed on a time-contingent basis as discussed in chapter 11. The use of antidepressants at this stage of treatment is often appropriate, depending upon symptom presentation. Depending on the severity of the chronic back-pain problem, investigating a full multidisciplinary-pain or functional-restoration program may be necessary.

Recurrent Acute Back Pain
Recurrent acute back pain may be one of the most common conditions that prompt people to seek periodic treatment. It is characterized by episodes of back pain of varying duration that are followed by essentially pain-free periods. The back pain can be of fluctuating intensities and can lead to varying levels of disability during the active phases. Occasionally the person can identify triggers to the back-pain episode, although we have seen many patients who report that they believe the episodes are unpredictable.

In dealing with recurrent acute back pain it is important to keep in mind that a vast majority of the population suffers from back pain at some time in their lifetime. Therefore back pain is a part of our normal human existence. The following will help effectively manage recurrent acute back-pain problems:

1. Become involved in a regular aerobic conditioning exercise program that is done at least three times per week. It appears that the exact type of exercise may

not be important, although it should contain aerobic, stretching, and strengthening components. Activities such as swimming, bicycling, and walking are excellent.

2. If you have been given a back-exercise program in the past, do it on a regular basis. In recurrent acute back-pain problems we discourage people from becoming dependent on a health care practitioner, as this tends to keep them in the sick role. We encourage patients to utilize their exercise program independently. In this way they develop effective self-management tools that help them whenever the back pain recurs.

3. Try to identify "triggers" to the occurrence of back pain. These might be either physically based or psychologically based.

4. The research is unclear as to whether good physical fitness can actually *prevent* recurrent acute back pain, though in our clinical experience it certainly seems to be the case. But there is growing research evidence that good physical conditioning can help decrease the frequency, intensity, and duration of these episodes when they do occur.

The biggest problem in managing recurrent acute back pain is compliance. Patients will generally be given the tools and recommendations to manage these problems, but follow-through is often quite poor. This is because the pain goes away and the person stops exercising.

Once you have developed a strategy to manage your back pain, be sure to follow through.

The bottom line is that you will get out of your own treatment program what you put into it.

PRINCIPLES FOR A BACK-CONDITIONING PROGRAM

The following sections discuss how to approach a conditioning program for your back-pain problem. The general principles include using the quota system, having an aerobic component to the program, and making sure that family and friends support you in the proper manner.

The Quota System

As mentioned, the quota system is a specialized approach to exercising (or to any activity for that manner) that involves working to a specific quota rather than being guided by the pain. It is important that this be done initially under the supervision of a physician and qualified physical therapist. The quota system can be applied for any type of exercise or activity that the patient wishes to increase.

In setting up a quota system for an exercise program the patient starts with what are called baseline measurements. In developing a baseline you exercise until pain or fatigue stops you over three consecutive sessions. An example of this might be doing repetitions of a strengthening exercise. You may only be able to do four repetitions on the first session, six repetitions on the second session, and five repetitions on the third session. Once the three baseline measures are taken, an average is then determined. In the example above, the average would be five repetitions for the particular exercise $(4 + 6 + 5 = 15$, divided by $3 = 5)$.

The initial quota is then set at 70 percent of the baseline average. Therefore you would begin the program for this particular exercise at an initial quota of three repetitions (70 percent of $4 = 2.8$, and round off to the next highest number). Setting the initial quota at 70 percent of the baseline average ensures that you will be successful in meeting the quota. Once the initial quota is established, you will do that number of repetitions regardless of the pain. The same type of quota can be set for such diverse things as walking distance, swimming distance, amount of time on a stationary bicycle, and any exercise that involves repetitions. A baseline measure is always taken over three or four sessions and then 70 percent of the average constitutes the initial quota. We usually recommend that the exercise program be done twice per day. The specifics of your particular program will be guided by your doctor.

An example of a completed quota progress record can be seen in figure 9-1, with a blank record for your own use in figure 9-2.

In this progress record, the activity is charted in two places: in the upper two boxes labeled "quota" and on the large graph, the axes of which are labeled "repetitions" and "session number." This gives a visual record of progress as well as the quota that is required for the specific exercise session. Note that in the upper charts of figure 9-1 there are "target" and "actual" headings under "quota." These are used to document your quota target for the exercise and the actual amount of the exercise done for that session. The quota system forces the exercise program to include a pacing component.

A question that must always be dealt with is how rapidly to increase the quotas. This is usually determined by the supervising doctor or physical therapist and will depend on the type of exercise as well as how chronic the back-pain problem has been. In addition the therapist will take into account how deconditioned the patient has become. Figure 9-1 is an example of a quota progress record completed for walking distance. As can be seen, the patient initially started out being able to walk an average of two city blocks (the baseline was the average of one, two, and three blocks). The patient decided to set the quotas for increase at a rate of one block every sixth session. Since the patient was walking twice a day, this translates into increasing the walking distance one block every three days. As can be seen, the walking distance increased significantly using the quota system. This program was done in conjunction with a variety of other exercises on a twice-per-day basis.

A quota progress record should be established for each exercise that is being done. Goals for each session are established from the beginning of the exercise program and the patient is progressed through the exercise program according to this pre-

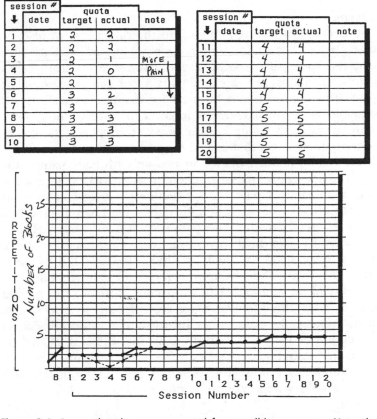

Figure 9-1. A completed progress record for a walking program. Note the quotas that have been set as goals and the actual distance walked for each session.

determined plan. Quotas can be adjusted slightly if there happens to be an acute exacerbation of pain. An example of this can be seen in the completed progress record in figure 9-1. In this example the patient did experience an acute exacerbation, which caused a significant decrease in the activity. The quotas were reestablished after the exacerbation, and again the patient began progressing toward increasing his walking distance.

Pacing

The concept of pacing is built into the quota system of exercise. Pacing is a technique for approaching any activity such that the back pain is kept under reasonable control. Pacing involves a gradual increase in activity according to a systematic plan. This approach can be used for exercise as well as any other activity. For instance it might also involve doing some activity and then taking regular breaks throughout the day to prevent acute exacerbations of the back pain.

A common pattern we see in people with back pain is the "overdo and crash" pattern, whereby the patient begins a day with minimal back pain and subsequently engages in so many activities that he or she is literally in bed with pain for the two or three days following. This pattern will then cycle such that the patient is continually overdoing activities when he or she begins to feel good and then "crashing" for several days thereafter. This is an unhealthy approach to back-pain rehabilitation and should be replaced with a "pacing" format. The patient would "pace" his activities regardless of how he is feeling in order to keep the pain under relatively good control. Pacing should not be confused with the concept of "being guided by the pain." Pacing encourages a reasonable amount of activity and exercise, not more and not less. The patient must attempt to do activities and exercise each day while pacing him- or herself.

Aerobic Conditioning

One component of a good exercise program for back pain must be aerobic conditioning. This should also initially be supervised by a physician or qualified physical therapist. Aerobic conditioning exercises are those that result in an increase in the uptake and utilization of oxygen. Actual aerobic conditioning occurs when the heart rate reaches a certain level and is

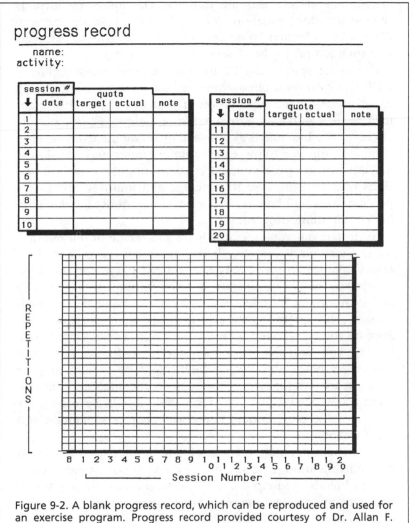

Figure 9-2. A blank progress record, which can be reproduced and used for an exercise program. Progress record provided courtesy of Dr. Allan F. Chino.

maintained at that level for a specific period of time. A rough estimate of a person's "target" heart rate for aerobic conditioning is the following: Subtract your age from 220 and then take

70 percent of the resulting number. The following formula represents this equation for a forty-five-year-old person: $220 - 45 = 175$, then 70 percent of $175 = 123$ (the target heart rate rounded off to the nearest whole number).

The quota system can be used for aerobic conditioning as well. First you must choose one or more aerobic conditioning exercises under the supervision of your physician. This might include such activities as brisk walking, swimming, or a stationary bike. The baseline is established by doing the exercise until you must stop due to increased pain or fatigue and you should *not* attempt to "push yourself." After doing three or four sessions of a baseline take the average and multiply this by 70 percent. This will give you your beginning quota for the aerobic conditioning program.

For instance if you can initially do an average of ten minutes on the stationary bicycle, then your initial quota would be seven minutes to start. A typical quota system for this type of exercise would be to start at seven minutes twice per day and increase the bicycle sessions by one minute every fourth session. This quota system will gradually increase your tolerance on the bicycle and increase the amount of aerobic conditioning you are able to obtain. You would do this until reaching a reasonable goal, which might be getting to your target heart rate for twenty minutes on the stationary bicycle three times per week. A similar system should be set up for other aerobic conditioning exercises, such as swimming and brisk walking.

Aerobic conditioning is an absolutely essential part of a back-pain rehabilitation program, not only for its conditioning component but also to help decrease stress, increase the fluidity of your movements, and decrease your overall pain.

Family, Friends, and Exercise

The last aspect of an exercise program is your psychosocial environment, which includes family, friends, and work associates. The psychosocial environment is an important element in any back-pain rehabilitation program. Consider the following case example, which is not uncommon in patients with back pain:

> A forty-six-year-old woman had undergone three previous spine surgeries. She had a developed chronic back-pain syndrome and was attempting to increase her functioning through many of the principles presented in this book. As she started to attempt more activities, she noticed that her husband would make comments such as "why don't you take it easy," "you shouldn't be doing that," and "you need to get more rest." She noticed that he was becoming overly protective and would often express to her that attempting to increase activities would certainly lead to injury. She noticed a similar reaction from many of her friends who knew she had a long-standing back-pain problem.

In this situation the patient's family and friends misunderstood her back-pain problem and the importance of the rehabilitation approach. The patient was instructed to educate them as to the importance of a quota-system-based increase in exercise and activity. She was also instructed to give them specific guidelines not to respond to her pain behaviors and to encourage her for any increase in activity that was observed. This example underscores that guidelines are needed in terms of dealing with family and friends when embarking on an exercise program or increasing one's activities. Specific guidelines are as follows:

- Educate your family and friends that increasing activities will not result in any harm and that it is the most healthy thing you can do for your back pain.

- Instruct them not to respond to pain behaviors but rather to provide encouragement for increasing activities or exercise.

- Tell as many people as possible of your plan to increase activities and of your exercise program. This type of public commitment will ensure that you follow through with your quota-based exercise conditioning program.

• One good way to ensure that you follow through with your exercise program is to get an "exercise buddy" (a family member or friend). Set up a regular schedule, and exercise in pairs. Then if one of you attempts to cancel out on a specific exercise session, you will need to be held accountable to your exercise partner.

EXERCISES FOR BACK PAIN

There are innumerable exercise approaches to back pain and it is beyond the scope and purpose of this book to present them. The findings of the AHCPR expert panel suggest the following general guidelines related to exercise:

• Low-stress exercise can prevent debilitation due to inactivity during the first month of back symptoms. In addition, beginning exercise at this early stage can help return you to your highest possible level of functioning.

• Aerobic (endurance) exercise programs that minimally stress the back can be started in the first two weeks of acute back pain for most patients.

• Conditioning exercises for the trunk muscles (gradually increased according to the quota method) are helpful, usually starting after the first two weeks of symptoms.

• High-tech back machines do not appear to provide benefit over traditional exercise in the treatment of acute back problems.

Your diagnosis and whether you have acute, subacute, chronic, or recurrent acute back-pain problems will determine which exercise program your doctor and/or physical therapist might recommend. It is important to be compliant in doing the exercises regularly and to use the quota-system approach.

SUMMARY OF THE CONDITIONING APPROACH

The following principles summarize how an exercise program should be managed:

1. Depending on your situation, you may need to check with your physician prior to beginning any type of exercise program.
2. A back exercise program can often be given to you by your family physician. If your back pain has persisted, or if you suffer from recurrent acute back pain, it may be most useful to begin a structured back exercise program under the supervision of a physician and physical therapist, or exercise physiologist.
3. It is always appropriate to stretch prior to exercising.
4. Include an aerobic component in your exercise program.
5. You should use "pacing" in terms of increasing the aggressiveness of your exercise program and general functioning. Many people will attempt to do too much too fast, which can result in an exacerbation and can increase the likelihood that you will not follow through on exercise. You should pace yourself and build the duration and intensity of the exercises according to a reasonable schedule.
6. Use the quota system and set goals for each exercise you are doing. This will ensure that you pace yourself. Also keep a progress record similar to that seen in figure 9-1 for each exercise in your program.
7. Do not be surprised if you experience a mild or moderate increase in pain in the initial stages of your reconditioning program. This is not uncommon and is most often related to the disuse syndrome. Do not be afraid of the pain.
8. Develop a system for yourself that will increase your compliance. This might involve exercising with a partner, developing a regular schedule for yourself, and rewarding yourself for completing a structured exercise program for a specified amount of time. We have found

that the biggest problem with a reconditioning program is noncompliance.

9. Talk to family and friends about how they can help you with your exercise program. Make a public commitment to the program.

CHAPTER 10

CONTROVERSIAL MEDICAL TREATMENTS FOR CHRONIC BACK PAIN AND THE FAILED-BACK-SURGERY SYNDROME

As we learned in the chapter discussing diagnosis, the chronic back-pain syndrome (CBPS) and the failed-back-surgery syndrome (FBSS) can be very debilitating for the patient and extremely difficult to treat. As you will recall, the chronic pain syndrome involves not only the continuation of the pain but many other secondary symptoms that have become part of the problem. The failed-back-surgery syndrome can occur for many reasons, but it is primarily a condition in which one or more back surgeries have been attempted but were not successful. Often the surgeons will say that the surgery was a "technical success," but the patient will report that the symptoms remain the same. In the failed-surgery syndrome, further surgery is most often not indicated and other treatment approaches are recommended.

These conditions are almost always best treated using a multidisciplinary rehabilitation approach because of the many factors that are affecting the pain and functioning (tissue damage, deconditioning, depression and anxiety, and substance abuse, among others; see figure 6-1). If all of the aspects of the condition are not treated simultaneously, the likelihood of improvement is minimal.

In response to these most-difficult-to-treat conditions, a number of treatment approaches have been developed. In our opinion, as well as in the opinion of most of the leaders in the field, these approaches continue to be controversial. They are probably appropriate for a very, very, very small percentage of patients with chronic back pain or failed-surgery syndrome. The most appropriate treatment is a multidisciplinary rehabilitation intervention such as the pain centers and functional-restoration programs described in chapter 8.

There are three primary controversial medical treatments that have been recommended for the treatment of CBPS and FBSS. These are chronic opioid therapy, dorsal column stimulation, and intraspinal drug infusion therapy. We are presenting the most current information on these techniques, as you might be advised to look into such treatments depending upon your back-pain condition and the orientation of the doctors you are working with. This information will help you become an informed consumer and help keep you from undergoing a technique that is not appropriate in your case.

CHRONIC OPIOID THERAPY FOR BACK PAIN

Chronic opioid therapy for back pain refers to the long-term administration of pain medicines (such as opiates; e.g., morphine) to patients with chronic back pain. This approach is highly controversial and has typically been rejected in the United States primarily due to fears of addiction, side effects, physical dependence, and tolerance. There are some physicians and researchers who feel that long-term use of opiates in very select patients with back pain can be an appropriate treatment. Again, we are presenting this approach for informational purposes only and would generally not suggest such an approach.

Dr. Russell Portenoy is probably best known for his research and interest in this area. He feels that there is a subpopulation of pain patients who are able to obtain at least partial pain relief from chronic opioid therapy without the development of toxicity or significant tolerance. He states that substance abuse behaviors may occur, but that these are uncommon if the patients are highly selected. Patients with a history of substance abuse tend to be at risk for developing problems in this regard. The most common physical side effects of long-term pain-medicine use seems to be persistent constipation, insomnia, and decreased sexual function. In addition there may be cognitive difficulties (trouble thinking clearly or focusing) and sedation initially, but it appears that these effects tend to diminish over time, although some patients do report continuing "mental clouding" sufficient to impair functioning.

In pursuing such a treatment approach with chronic non-cancer-pain patients (such as back pain), Dr. Portenoy has proposed guidelines for patient selection and evaluation of the treatment. The ones relevant to this discussion are as follows:

1. Chronic opioid therapy should be considered only after all other reasonable attempts at pain control have failed.
2. Any history of substance abuse should preclude this type of approach.
3. A single practitioner (doctor) should take primary responsibility for this treatment.
4. Patients must receive adequate informed consent prior to starting the treatment.
5. Doses should be given on a time-contingent, around-the-clock, basis (see chapter 11 for a discussion of how to take pain medicine).
6. The patient should obtain at least partial pain relief at relatively low initial doses. If this is not seen, then this type of treatment is probably not appropriate.
7. This type of approach should be done in conjunction with treatments that emphasize increases in physical and social function concomitantly.
8. Most patients should be seen on at least a monthly basis.
9. Evidence of drug hoarding, getting drugs from other doctors, uncontrolled escalation in doses, or other problem behaviors should result in discontinuation of the program.

Based on our experience, we feel that very few patients might be appropriate for this type of approach. Patient selection is critical, as is working with a physician who is knowledgeable of this type of treatment. Certainly, prior to utilizing this kind of approach, a behavioral/psychological approach to pain management including physical and mental reconditioning programs should be attempted. Even if these are not entirely successful, they should be continued with the long-term pain-medication program as Dr. Portenoy suggests in number 7 above.

We have seen many patients who are receiving long-term pain-medication therapy that are either completely inappropriate for this approach or who are doing it in an incorrect fashion. All aspects of such an approach as listed above must be adhered to in an ongoing manner. In addition, patients will often have unrealistic expectations about using opiates long-term, believing that "if my pain were gone, then I would resume my life." The chronic opioid therapy approach for back pain tends to reinforce this type of thinking, often to the exclusion of increasing functioning and improving other aspects of a person's life. Our preference is to recommend a multidisciplinary pain rehabilitation program that focuses on these issues rather than moving toward a chronic opioid approach.

SPINAL CORD STIMULATION

Spinal cord stimulation is a technique that was introduced more than twenty years ago as a reversible, nondestructive method for the management of chronic, intractable pain. Spinal cord stimulation is also termed dorsal column stimulation (DCS), which is descriptive of the technique. In the simplest of terms, a set of electrodes is surgically placed along the dorsal nerve fibers of the spinal cord in the lower back in order to block pain impulses passing through that area.

The idea of spinal cord stimulation is based on the gate-control theory, which has been discussed previously. Basically the electrical stimulation provided by the stimulator causes a blockage of the pain impulses at the spinal cord level. This is similar to the rationale behind the TENS unit, which is discussed under the treatments chapter.

Dorsal column stimulation is primarily appropriate as a last resort to treat the failed-back-surgery syndrome and/or arachnoiditis (see chapter 6). It has also been used for nerve-root injuries that have not responded to previously conservative treatments and/or corrective surgeries. It is generally agreed that dorsal column stimulation is only considered after all conservative therapies have been exhausted, and only in patients who have been screened very carefully in a variety of ways.

Patients who might be appropriate for dorsal column stimulators have the following characteristics:

1. The pain from a spine problem is primarily in one or both legs. The pain in the legs must be the primary complaint. Dorsal column stimulation is not appropriate where lower back pain is the sole complaint.
2. Any disease process is "static" (essentially not changing).
3. The pain is primarily neuropathic and radicular in nature (due to a nerve problem and "radiating" from the lower back to the legs).
4. The pain is primarily experienced as "burning, stinging, tingling, and radiating."
5. The patient has failed all previous attempts at conservative treatments, which would include such things as physical therapy, psychological interventions, nerve blocks, medication management, and multidisciplinary rehabilitation.
6. The patient's complaints are consistent with physical findings.

If these criteria are met, the patient still may or may not be appropriate for a trial of dorsal column stimulation. The patient's selection is the critical variable in this procedure. Many surgeons will have the attitude of "giving it a try when all else fails" and not using appropriate screening techniques. Under these conditions there are certain to be a high percentage of failures. As discussed above, the primary group for which dorsal column stimulators are possibly recommended is that of the failed-back-surgery syndrome. Further, even in this group a very small percentage will meet the criteria listed above in addition to the screening procedures we are about to discuss.

Prior to consideration for this type of treatment, a multidisciplinary evaluation is essential. This should involve an evaluation from such professionals as the surgeon, an internist, and a psychologist or psychiatrist. Patients who are not appropriate for consideration of dorsal column stimulation would include those patients who do not meet the above criteria. In addition if the patient does meet these criteria, he or she should *not* show any of the following:

1. Symptoms (pain or other complaints) that do not match physical findings or that show nonphysiological signs and symptoms. This would include evidence of symptom amplification, which is discussed in chapter 14.
2. Serious drug-seeking behavior, which would include elements of addiction.
3. Lower back pain as the sole complaint.
4. Lack of motivation in attempting this approach in addition to addressing other aspects of the chronic pain syndrome of FBSS.
5. Psychological or emotional factors that would preclude a successful response.

If the surgeon is rigorous in adhering to the aforementioned screening criteria, the number of patients that are appropriate for consideration of dorsal column stimulation is quite small.

Once a patient reaches this stage of consideration and has passed all of the screening criteria, a temporary electrode is placed to determine whether dorsal column stimulation might be effective. The patient's response to the temporary electrode placement will determine whether there will be actual implantation of a permanent device. Surgeons will differ as to the duration of the test phase and the amount of pain relief they require before consideration of permanent implantation.

The average length of the test phase for the temporary electrode is generally accepted to be approximately two to three days, although some surgeons will require a test phase of up to two months. The generally accepted standard for pain relief is usually 50 to 70 percent reduction with the temporary electrode. It appears that a minimum criterion of 50 percent relief is average.

If you are being considered for dorsal column stimulation, it is important to be truthful with your physician as to the amount of pain relief actually experienced during the test phase. Some studies indicate that up to 22 percent of patients will report they are experiencing pain relief when they are not. This is done in an attempt to get the permanent device. Since the test phase predicts how well the device will work, not being truthful leads to unnecessary surgery and treatment failure.

Even with a good screening and an adequate response to the test phase and permanent implantation, "tolerance" to the system can develop in some patients (about 25 percent), resulting in a gradual decline in pain relief. This tolerance tends to occur within the first four years after implantation, with the greatest decline in pain control during the first two years. If the system is still working after four years, the long-term prognosis for sustained pain relief is good.

Complications of spinal cord stimulation treatment include such things as displacement of the electrode or electrode movement, infection, the electrode fracturing, battery depletion, an electrical "leak," or a cerebral spinal fluid leak. These complications are quite rare and are easily addressed.

INTRASPINAL DRUG INFUSION THERAPY

Many patients with the failed-back-surgery syndrome will complain primarily of back pain rather than pain radiating down one or both legs. As discussed previously, the dorsal column stimulator technique should only be considered in patients who have leg pain as the primary complaint. Pain that is primarily in the lower back is not responsive to dorsal column stimulator therapy.

Intraspinal drug infusion therapy involves surgically implanting in the body a "pump system" through which pain medicine is delivered by a small tube (catheter) directly into a specific area of the spine. The rationale behind this approach is that much less pain medicine is required for the relief of back pain if the medicine is delivered directly to the spine. When pain medicines are taken orally, their effects are systemic (which means "throughout the body") and only a fraction of the medicine is actually working where it is needed. The intraspinal drug infusion method is purported to make the medicine more effective and with less side effects.

The procedure for consideration of an implanted pump system is very similar to that of consideration for dorsal column stimulation. Patients who are considered for this type of procedure are generally those who have a failed-back-surgery syndrome or chronic back pain in which all previous treatments have failed. Clinical criteria for consideration usually include the following:

1. Pain primarily in the lower back and buttocks, with only minimal radiation down one or both legs.
2. Multiple pain sites in the lower back and buttocks with a complaint of "diffuse pain."
3. Pain that is not described primarily as nerve pain.
4. The patient has not responded to all other available conservative treatments including medications, physical therapy, nerve blocks, or behavioral/psychological interventions.

If the patient meets these criteria, there are additional screening parameters that must also be addressed. Again this is a process that is similar to that of evaluation for dorsal column stimulation. The screening criteria that would preclude patients are as follows:

1. Symptoms (pain or other complaints) that do not match physical findings or that show nonphysiological signs and symptoms. This would include evidence of symptom amplification, which is discussed in chapter 14.
2. Serious drug-seeking behavior, which would include elements of addiction.
3. Leg pain (versus back pain) as the sole complaint.
4. Lack of motivation to attempt such an approach in addition to addressing other aspects of the chronic pain syndrome of FBSS.
5. Psychological or emotional factors that preclude a successful response.

If a patient meets all the appropriate criteria, a test phase is done before considering a fully implantable pump system. In the test phase the pump is outside the body with a catheter delivering medicine to a spine area. The test phase will generally be for two to three days with a 50 percent relief criterion. Of course it is important to be truthful during this phase, as it is predictive of the success of the permanently implanted device.

The permanently implanted system involves placing a small reservoir (the pump) under the skin; this pump has a tube that delivers the pain medicine to the spine. The reservoir needs to be refilled approximately every two weeks by placing a needle through the skin into the reservoir pump and filling it with more pain medicine. Drug doses must be carefully selected to avoid oversedation and all of the side effects associated with opioid use.

Complications related to intraspinal morphine pump delivery systems include infection, contamination of the pump reservoir, cerebral spinal fluid leak, postspinal headache, mechanical pump failure, mechanical catheter failure, and side effects to the medication.

Problems with this approach include the facts that the reservoir must be filled every one to three weeks, that there may be the need for gradually increasing doses of the medication, which defeats its purpose, and that many patients are not comfortable with having this device in their body.

The morphine pump procedure remains controversial, and patients should have attempted absolutely all other treatment approaches prior to considering it. In addition psychological evaluation should be done prior to this therapy.

When all of the foregoing factors are considered, in our opinion there will be very few patients who are appropriate either for intraspinal morphine pump systems or for dorsal column stimulator approaches.

SUMMARY AND CONCLUSIONS

There are several key points that are common to all three of the controversial approaches described above. If you have been recommended for any of these approaches, careful consideration of these and all factors should be made by you and by your doctor(s).

First, all of these treatment approaches are essentially "end-stage," which means that one criterion for consideration is that nothing else has worked. A *credible* multidisciplinary rehabilitation approach should have been attempted prior to consideration. We have seen many patients who state they have gone through such a multidisciplinary program when in fact they have not. Many programs will purport to offer a comprehensive "multidisciplinary" approach even though they do not. You and your doctor should very carefully assess the type and quality of previous treatments you have had in addition to discussing why the previous treatments (including the multidisciplinary rehabilitation) did not work. Many factors that caused that treatment not to work (e.g., lack of motivation, emotional factors, drug-seeking behavior, litigation issues) might cause the controversial measures to be unsuccessful.

Second, your doctor should be adhering to the selection criteria as presented in this book (which represents the agreed-upon approach in the research literature). There are great pressures that can come to bear causing a doctor to recommend a controversial approach when it is not appropriate and has a low probability of success. One pressure is financial. The surgeons are heavily marketed by the companies that produce these units. The two surgical procedures (spinal stimulators and implantable pumps) are very costly and can be high-income producers for certain surgical practices.

Third is the attitude of "nothing else has worked, why not give it a try," which is often shared by both patient and doctor. This is not a good reason to forgo the screening process. If you have a low probability of success for one of these treatments, it will set you up for yet another treatment "failure," which can lead to a greater sense of hopelessness, depression, and anxiety. This in turn will make your overall condition worse. In addition you will be suffering from increased financial stress due to the costs either to you or to your insurance company. Even in situations where the costs are being paid by a third party, if the treatment is unsuccessful, they are going to be unlikely to approve any further treatments.

We believe it is important for patients to be well educated and informed regarding the nature of these procedures. If any of the above procedures are recommended, you should seriously consider obtaining a second opinion from a doctor with a rehabilitation focus.

CHAPTER 11

MEDICATIONS FOR BACK PAIN: WHAT YOU NEED TO KNOW

Let's begin by saying that back pain does not necessarily require medication in its treatment. This is a decision to be reached by you and your doctor. This chapter will give you a good understanding about the medicines used in the treatment of back pain. In addition it will give you information about how these medicines should be taken and will discuss mistakes often made in the use of these medicines.

Traditional medicine will often look to medicating back-pain suffering without providing other treatments (e.g., aggressive conditioning, relaxation training, and mind-body approaches), which are more likely to have long-term benefit. In virtually all cases of back pain, if a decision is made to use medication, it should be done in conjunction with a treatment plan including other approaches. Medications can be useful as a helpful adjunct in decreasing pain, reducing inflammation, and relieving muscle spasm.

The few exceptions in which medication is clearly indicated for the treatment of back pain include infections, severe osteoporosis, rare tumors, and acute spinal cord compression. As this subset represents a very small percentage of back-pain sufferers, we will not discuss the roles of individual medications for each of these cases.

When discussing the more common medications we see used on a daily basis for the majority of back-pain sufferers, we can divide them into six general categories, as follows:

- Anti-inflammatories
- Muscle relaxants

- Analgesics
- Antidepressants
- Antianxiety agents
- Sedatives

These medications, used individually and in combinations, may accelerate the healing process and facilitate the use of other approaches while keeping the patient more comfortable.

ANTI-INFLAMMATORIES

Anti-inflammatories are a class of medications that, as their name implies, have the purpose of reducing inflammation. Inflammation can also be thought of as a "swelling" and includes a process whereby local chemical irritants are released from the involved tissue. These chemicals have several effects on the surrounding tissue, including altering the normal patterns of blood flow and irritating the nerve endings, which carry pain sensation.

As an example, when you suffer from a bruise, you will see a black-and-blue mark, or bump on the skin, including swelling. This happens because of a local inflammatory reaction in which various chemicals are released, causing leakage of fluid into the local area, irritation of nerve endings, and changes in blood flow.

The chemicals released during the inflammatory process include prostaglandins, which have an ability to stimulate various cells associated with the inflammatory process. If not brought under control, this inflammatory process can persist and impede healing, as well as being painful. Anti-inflammatories are directed at stopping the inflammatory process by inhibiting the production of prostaglandins.

One of the original anti-inflammatory drugs commonly used is aspirin. Besides reducing inflammation, aspirin also has the properties of being a painkiller and antifever medication. In many studies aspirin has been found to be as effective as other prescription medications for back pain. Although aspirin remains the first and most widely used of the anti-inflammatories, it can be associated with several side effects, which include gastrointestinal upset, ulcers, and increased bleeding tendencies, among others. Using enteric-coated forms of aspirin to protect the GI tract can help with some of these side effects. Certainly aspirin compounds should be a first line of medication treatment for back pain.

There has been a rapid proliferation in the development of various classes of anti-inflammatory agents. All of these have certain pharmacologic similarities in that they inhibit the synthesis of prostaglandins. The most commonly known anti-inflammatories presently used in the United States, aside from aspirin, include ibuprofen (Motrin and Advil) and naproxen (Naprosyn and Aleve). People use these anti-inflammatories for everything from sports injuries to menstrual cramps to headaches.

With regard to back pain, there are various factors to be considered when evaluating whether to use anti-inflammatories. Many types of back pain are considered to have an inflammatory component, such as muscle sprain-strains and injuries to the soft tissues. These injuries are usually associated with an excessive lifting, twisting, or bending beyond the normal capacity of the muscles, tendons, and ligaments. In addition new research continues to emphasize the inflammatory component as a source of pain in degenerative disc disease, as well as in certain types of bulging and herniated discs. Finally, there are certain types of rare arthritic conditions in the spine that are known to have an inflammatory component. All of these conditions may be appropriate for the use of anti-inflammatories.

Because anti-inflammatories can cause nausea and GI upset, the medication should only be taken with meals. Anti-inflammatories can also increase bleeding time, which slows down blood clot formation and increases the possibility of bruising. Less common side effects include tinnitus (ringing in the ears), light-headedness, and gastritis. Many of the anti-inflammatories are metabolized primarily by the kidneys and some by the liver, so chronic use may lead to some damage to these organs. The main reasons not to use anti-inflammatories include ulcer disease and bleeding problems. Anti-inflammatories should be prescribed on a regular dosing schedule for most of the above-mentioned conditions and usually continued for approximately two weeks. This allows for establishment and maintenance of a therapeutic blood level. Let's discuss ibuprofen as an example, as it is one of the most commonly prescribed nonsteroidal anti-inflammatory drugs (NSAID). A typical prescription should read as follows:

Ibuprofen, 400 mg four times per day with meals for two weeks on a regular schedule. This dosage can be increased to either 600 or 800 mg four times per day with meals assuming that there are no intolerable side effects.

It should be noted that patients will often have a tendency to discontinue the use of their anti-inflammatories within the first couple of days of treatment when they start to feel better. We often see a recurrence of symptoms from this discontinuation of the anti-inflammatory. The initial course should usually be continued for approximately two weeks, but certainly as prescribed by the treating physician. As the physician often has a goal of obtaining a certain blood level of medication when prescribing it, the patient should be cautioned to discuss with him or her any desire to stop the medication prematurely or to change the dosage, even if the symptoms seem to have disappeared. Also anti-inflammatories should usually be used on a time-limited basis due to the side effects listed above.

These medications serve as an adjunct to the natural healing powers of the body and should never be considered as a substitute for proper exercise or used as a single form of treatment.

MUSCLE RELAXANTS

Muscle relaxants are usually prescribed with the goal of reducing muscle spasm and should take a much more limited role in treating back pain than anti-inflammatories. They are indicated only when muscle spasm is *clearly* a prominent feature of the back-pain sufferer's problem.

How muscle relaxants work remains somewhat controversial. Many of these medications are known to work through the central nervous system (the brain) and thereby secondarily relax the muscles by relaxing the brain. There are several muscle relaxants that appear to work directly on the cells of the muscle itself by decreasing the "hypercontractual state" (overcontracted or in spasm). However, these also have known effects on the central nervous system.

Among the more commonly prescribed muscle relaxants we see in use today in back-pain patients are Valium, Soma, Robaxin, and Flexeril. As all of these are known to have effects on the brain, including a slowing of overall mental functioning and sedation, their use should be limited to one to two weeks, except in very exceptional cases as recommended by a physician. You should not take muscle relaxants when operating heavy machinery or driving, and never mix them with alcohol.

Muscle relaxants are often prescribed for use in the evenings in the early phases of acute back pain associated with muscle spasms to help the patient sleep. It is important to avoid becoming dependent on these muscle relaxants as a sleep medication, as they might have a tendency to disturb sleep patterns in the long run. In addition long-term use of these medications may potentially promote symptoms of depression.

Many muscle relaxants (most notably Valium) also play a role in reducing anxiety through their effects on the brain. Although this might be helpful for a short period of time in patients with acute severe back pain, they should be avoided for long-term use, as there is a tendency toward addiction. In addition they should general not be prescribed if it becomes clear that they are being used for anxiety and agitation rather than spasm.

Unlike nonsteroidal anti-inflammatories, it can be appropriate to utilize muscle relaxants on an as-needed basis in the early course of treatment. If the spasm is severe and not responding to ice, heat, or stretching, then muscle relaxants can be used as an adjunct for short-term relief. They should never be used as a substitute for these other methods of reducing spasm.

An interesting point to consider is that muscle relaxants are often the only medications to afford relief in patients with stress-related back pain. Muscle relaxants work so well in this group because they help reduce anxiety and "relax the brain," thereby reducing the stress that is causing the pain. Muscle spasm may not even be present in these cases.

The most common side effects of muscle relaxants, as previously stated, relate to their depressant effects on the central nervous system. Dependency on the medication is the other major concern in view of their role in reducing anxiety, helping with sleep, and causing somewhat of a euphoric state in some individuals. Dosages of these medications vary significantly and should be discussed with your treating physician as to the specific indications.

In summary, the role of muscle relaxants should be quite limited to cases where muscle spasm is a well-defined component that is not responding to physical interventions, such as ice, heat, and stretching. For chronic spasms biofeedback and relaxation training would be more appropriate. Chronic use of muscle relaxants is not indicated for back pain. Some specialists will rarely use muscle relaxants for two reasons. First, there is controversy as to whether muscle spasm is even significant in back pain. Second, the muscle tension, if it is present, may actually serve a protective function. These reasons, as well as those listed above, underscore that

> **Muscle relaxants should only be used in clear cases of muscle spasm when other modalities have not been effective and only on a time-limited basis.**

ANALGESICS (PAINKILLERS)

Analgesics, or painkillers, are among the most commonly used medications for back pain. They are also the most over-prescribed and inappropriately used medications in this area. Their purpose is strictly for pain relief, usually in the short term, except in rare cases of chronic back pain with progressive underlying disease, such as cancer.

Analgesics have a broad range of intensity ranging from the mild over-the-counter preparations (aspirin and Tylenol, for example) to the very strong narcotics, such as morphine. It should be noted here that many of the nonsteroidal anti-inflammatories, such as ibuprofen and aspirin, have analgesic properties that can provide pain relief as well as reduce inflammation.

Among the more commonly prescribed analgesics that are not also anti-inflammatories are codeine and drugs derived from codeine. These include such medicines as Tylenol with codeine, hydrocodone (Vicodin), oxycodone (Percodan), and dihydrocodeine. Often these medicines have a narcotic or synthetic narcotic component combined with Tylenol or aspirin.

These types of medicines are generally indicated only in the early acute phases of severe back pain. As with the other medicines discussed, they should be used in addition to other methods for pain relief (limited bed rest, ice, heat, etc.). It is important to note here that these stronger analgesics are generally prescribed on an "as-needed" basis, for instance, "Take one or two tablets as needed every four to six hours for pain." This is appropriate for short-term acute pain, though when given directions in this manner, patients will often try to wait until the pain is unbearable before taking the analgesic. This is often due to a fear of addiction and dependence. At that point the pain is so severe that the medication will have a lessened effect. Then the person is likely to take more (e.g., three tablets) to get the pain under control. This sets up a pattern of medication use that will result in less pain relief and higher levels of pain while taking more medicine!

When taking the analgesic on an as-needed basis in the acute phases of back pain, it is important to use the medicine to help prevent the pain from building up rather than "toughing it out." This will result in less pain medicine use overall and better pain control. You can be more comfortable using this approach if you know that the research shows that people who use pain medicines in this manner for acute back pain do not become "addicts" unless there are issues unrelated to the pain (e.g., a history of substance abuse).

Strong analgesics should be used in a time-limited fashion and always in conjunction with other treatment approaches. The most common side effects seen with narcotic analgesics include nausea, constipation, lethargy, decreased mental functioning, irritability, and sedation. Tylenol, the most widely used analgesic today, can cause liver damage if taken in exceedingly high doses or over very long periods of time. Many of the narcotic analgesics are combined with either Tylenol or aspirin, so both liver and kidney function might need to be monitored in patients using these medications over a longer period.

Many chronic back-pain sufferers have been prescribed analgesics for long-term use. There are several problems with the rationale of long-term analgesic use for back pain. In discussing these medicines we need to define the terms *tolerance, dependence,* and *addiction.*

A well-known pharmacologic property of all the narcotic analgesics is known as *tolerance.* This means that the body gets used to the effect of the medication and needs a steadily increasing dose over time to give the same level of pain relief. Tolerance occurs at a chemical level in the body primarily through the liver producing more enzymes to neutralize the effects of the medicine. As the dose goes up over time, we also see increased side effects (nausea, constipation, sedation, problems with thinking, etc.), including dependence and the possibility of addiction. Some doctors believe that a certain level of narcotic can be reached for pain control and stabilized for long-term use. However, we have generally found that the amount needed for back-pain control continues to rise over time with increasing side effects and the ultimate need for detoxification.

Dependence on a medication means that if it were suddenly stopped, withdrawal symptoms would appear. This might include such things as tremors, cramps, agitation, sleep disruption, and diarrhea. One might also notice an increase in the pain over the short term. Dependence is also related to chemical events in the body similar to the process of tolerance.

Addiction is a psychological craving for the medication. It includes aspects of tolerance and dependency due to the chemical events associated with long-term use. It should be noted that although addiction includes tolerance and dependence, the reverse is not necessarily true. One can show tolerance and dependence without showing addiction. In fact addiction is a well-known, although relatively rare, occurrence in patients using narcotics for pain relief.

Dr. Richard Sternbach has identified how tolerance and dependence on pain medicine can actually lead to higher levels of pain. Patients who have attained higher levels of pain-medicine use will occasionally attempt to decrease their use. When they do attempt this decrease, withdrawal symptoms occur, the most prominent of which is usually an increase in pain. The patient will state that he or she does not have a "craving" for the medication except to relieve the pain. This increase in pain, in addition to the lack of craving, is then used as a rationale for the patient (and the patient's doctor) to once again increase the analgesic use, stopping the withdrawal symptoms, and decreasing the pain. This pattern will only lead to higher levels of pain, dependence, and tolerance.

Dr. Sternbach has identified this phenomenon as a "conditioned pain response." In this process, at the early stages of pain medication use you wait until the back pain is very severe before taking the medicine. The pain medicine results in a decrease in pain, which is a positive reinforcer. Anything that results in positive reinforcement is likely to be done again or to occur again. Therefore the next time you have pain, you are more likely to take a pain pill. This process continues until tolerance and dependence develop. When this occurs, the withdrawal symptom of increased pain is more likely to occur as the medication wears off. As Dr. Sternbach says, "The pain becomes more severe as a signal to replenish the supply of narcotics which the body has now come to need." This, then, becomes a conditioned pain response in which higher pain levels are reinforced by the pain medicine. It should be noted that this process is not related to imaginary pain or addictive behavior.

A significant controversy exists among medical professionals in determining the appropriate long-term use for narcotic analgesics in back pain. There is widespread acceptance that it is reasonable to use narcotic analgesics for pain relief in the short term when the patient has severe back pain and is unable to obtain relief by any other means. The acute phase would generally cover the first two to three weeks, although it may extend as far as six weeks from initial pain onset. The few diagnoses where there is fairly good acceptance for more long-term use of the narcotic analgesics include cancer pain, spinal infections (with accompanying antibiotic therapy), and fractures (often accompanied by bracing).

Among the most controversial areas in considering the use of narcotic analgesics is the diagnosis of failed-back-surgery syndrome. It is our opinion that there are very few patients for whom the long-term use of narcotic analgesics is appropriate. In these cases we certainly feel there is a strong need for an aggressive conservative pain-management program including physical exercises and cognitive behavioral therapy. Narcotic analgesics are occasionally utilized as an adjunct to this approach in order to maintain and maximize the patient's level of function. However, we have seen numerous patients with failed-back-surgery syndromes overcome their disabilities, as well as their chronic dependency on narcotic analgesics, by utilizing the mental approaches to pain control, as well as a structured physical conditioning program and other techniques.

Another diagnosis in which narcotics are used long-term is that of "chronic benign back pain." This is generally back pain of long duration in which identifiable structural pathology to explain the pain is not found. The use of narcotics in this diagnostic group is very controversial, and most physicians prefer other pain-control approaches.

Any analgesic taken long-term should be used on a "time-contingent" basis rather than "as-needed." On a time-contingent schedule the medication is taken on a fixed schedule rather than according to symptoms, regardless of the pain level. For instance the schedule might be one tablet every four hours. The idea behind this approach is to keep the pain-relieving effect constant, avoid the ups and downs of the as-needed approach, and prevent the conditioned pain response from occurring. It can also prevent severe pain episodes by catching the pain early.

In addition to the time-contingent approach, it is important to utilize the lowest level of pain medicine possible. This will help avoid tolerance and keep dependence from occurring, in addition to ameliorating the side effects of the medicine.

We have mentioned some of the problematic side effects of narcotic analgesics, including dependence, tolerance, and addiction. Overall, however, pure analgesics are considered by many to be relatively safe when used in a limited fashion. Also, newer research has shown that using these medicines for acute back pain on a time-limited basis does not create "addicts," as was previously believed. This has been determined by extensive research in the area of cancer-pain management, where narcotics are commonly utilized, often in fairly high dosages for long periods of time.

ANTIDEPRESSANTS

Antidepressants are playing an increasing role as a medication adjunct in the treatment of chronic back-pain problems. Extensive research is showing that certain antidepressant medications can provide pain relief in chronic back pain. It should be noted that this effect is seen even in patients who are not depressed. Therefore the pain relief appears to occur independent of the antidepressant effect.

Extensive research is presently being done to better understand the exact roles of antidepressants for pain management in a variety of conditions. Some of the most widely used antidepressants in the area of chronic back pain are as follows:

Imipramine (Tofranil)

Amitriptyline (Elavil)

Doxepin (Sinequan)

Nortriptyline (Pamelor)

Desipramine (Norpramine)

Clomipramine (Anafranil)

Trazadone (Desyrel)

Fluoxetine (Prozac)

Although the exact mechanism remains somewhat unclear as to how these medicines afford pain relief, they are considered to be helpful to various degrees in different patients. The antidepressants work by increasing the action of certain neurotransmitters (brain chemicals). As there is clearly a very intimate relationship between emotional states, brain chemistry, and pain, it is not surprising that these medications have shown such promise in many refractory cases of chronic back pain.

The choice of antidepressant medication will depend on the symptoms you are experiencing. Some of the antidepressants have sedative properties, while others have an energizing effect. In addition different antidepressants will affect different brain chemicals (serotonin and norepinephrine). Factors to be considered by you and your doctor in deciding to use these medicines will be presented below.

First, we must consider the role that antidepressants have in improving restful sleep in addition to decreasing pain. Many chronic back-pain patients, especially those with neuropathic (nerve) pain radiating down the legs, have great difficulty obtaining restful sleep. The sedative properties of some of the antidepressants can be very helpful in normalizing sleep patterns while at the same time playing a role in the reduction of pain. The antidepressants seem to provide better restful sleep and other positive benefits (e.g., pain relief) than sleeping medications.

Table 11-1. Dosage Ranges for Antidepressants When Used for Pain Versus Depression

Antidepressant	Dosage Range for Pain	Dosage Range for Depression
Norpramine	75 mg	75–200 mg
Pamelor	50–100 mg	75–150 mg
Sinequan	50–100 mg	150–300 mg
Tofranil	50–75 mg	150–300 mg
Elavil	25–150 mg	150–300 mg
Desyrel	unknown	150–400 mg
Prozac	unknown	20–80 mg

Second, the medicines are also sometimes intended to have some role in combating depression, which is commonly seen in varying degrees associated with chronic back-pain suffering. However, we should reiterate that even if the patient is not clinically depressed, there appears to be a property in many of the antidepressants that decreases pain. This pain-relief property occurs at dosage ranges much less than are used in the treatment of depression. For instance a typical dose of Elavil for chronic pain would be approximately 50 to 75 milligrams, whereas the antidepressant dose might typically be 100 to 150 milligrams or more. There are also many patients who seem to have a significant reduction of their pain and improvement in sleep with even lower doses of antidepressants. It should be noted that dosage ranges for pain and depression are different depending upon the antidepressant used. This is illustrated in table 11-1.

Although we commonly prescribe antidepressants in our practice, we clearly recognize them as an adjunct and attempt to limit their use to the short term. We use them in addition to other approaches including exercise and cognitive therapy.

Some of the newer antidepressants (e.g., Prozac, Zoloft, Paxil, and Effexor) are just now being researched and increasingly used in patients with chronic back pain. These medications are more specific in their actions on certain brain chemicals. Currently the most common and well known of these is Prozac. These antidepressants have not yet been extensively studied for their role in decreasing pain. Their use appears to be more limited to patients who have depression associated with chronic back pain. Future research will help clarify how to most effectively use these medicines in back pain.

Patients should be instructed that it is important to take the antidepressant medications as prescribed on a daily basis. These medicines are not taken on an as-needed basis, as it is important to obtain a proper blood level for them to be effective. Depending on the medication, it will either be taken every night before bed (for the more sedating) or every morning (for the more energizing).

Side effects will vary depending upon the medication used. Common side effects include dry mouth, blurred vision, constipation, urinary retention, sedation, and nausea, among others. Side effects will usually be experienced when starting antidepressant medication and dissipate after two to three weeks or sooner. You must help your doctor monitor side effects, as this will determine the dosage range and influence the choice of medication. Mild side effects at the beginning of treatment are generally to be expected, but all side effects should be reported to your doctor.

In addition the dosages of these medications frequently have to be adjusted and tailored to the individual patient. It may take up to several months to find both the proper dose and the proper antidepressant medication for an individual patient. Patients should communicate regularly with their physician and be well informed about changes in the doses and side effects. It is important not to get frustrated during this adjustment phase when trying antidepressant medications as an adjunct in controlling pain.

Many patients are concerned with becoming chronically dependent on these medications, as well as of the possibilities of long-term side effects. It should be understood that antidepressant medicines are not addictive, and tolerance in the sense of narcotic analgesics does not develop.

In prescribing these medications we will usually begin at the lowest starting dose and raise it until the therapeutic effect is seen. The rate of dosage increase will be guided by side effects. Subsequently it is generally our practice to taper these medications between three and twelve months after reaching their therapeutic level. At that point we like to have the patient employing more self-management techniques, such as relaxation procedures, meditation, biofeedback, and exercise as a substitute for these medications. We do, however, find certain cases where they are required for more long-term use and can be extremely helpful, especially where there is a chronic underlying depression. In these cases it is most appropriate to have a consultation with a physician who is familiar with both chronic pain and medication approaches to depression.

ANTIANXIETY AGENTS

Antianxiety agents are occasionally used in acute back pain for their role in decreasing anxiety and helping with sleep. The most widely used antianxiety agents are known as benzodiazepines, which include such medications as Valium, Ativan, Xanax, Tranxene, and Centrax. As discussed previously, Valium is also used as a muscle relaxant and most likely exerts the majority of its effect on the central nervous system. Many patients with stress-related back pain find antianxiety medications to be very helpful, although these clearly should not be used as a substitute for more independent stress- and pain-management techniques.

We generally discourage the use of these agents for anything but very short periods and in very specific cases. If the back pain is associated with a high degree of anxiety and agitation, these medications can be useful. As with the other medications, they should be used as part of a comprehensive approach to the back pain, on a time-limited basis.

There are certain patients with more severe anxiety disorders who also suffer from chronic back pain. These patients can require more long-term use of antianxiety medications when they are unable to respond to other interventions. The patient should be followed closely and regularly by a physician familiar with the long-term use of these medicines.

Common side effects of the benzodiazepines include drowsiness, sedation, and short-term memory loss, among others. Many of these are eliminated by adjusting the dose. In addition tolerance and dependence do develop when using these medications, just as in the case of pain medicines. Care should be taken to avoid alcohol while taking these medications. Also you should never abruptly stop taking benzodiazepines. The medications should be tapered under your doctor's guidance.

SEDATIVES/HYPNOTICS

Sedatives (also termed hypnotics) are used for sleep. There are a variety of medications classed in this group, but they generally include benzodiazepines (Dalmane, Restoril, Halcion), barbiturates (Amytal, Nembutal, Seconal), chloral derivatives (chloral hydrate), and antihistamines (Benadryl).

In using these medications one must first look at the reasons for sleep problems. If they are related to depression, then an antidepressant should be used. If they are related to anxiety, then an antianxiety agent should be used. If they are related to pain, then an analgesic or low-dose sedating antidepressant might be most appropriate. If none of these is the case, then consideration of a sedative may be appropriate.

In choosing a sedative the least addictive should be tried first. Using Benadryl (50 to 150 milligrams at bedtime) is a very good first choice. If that is ineffective, the benzodiazepines can provide a good sedative effect. These are relatively safe medicines and are the least disruptive to certain types of sleep patterns. The use of barbiturates has fallen into disfavor due to the potential for abuse and the availability of the much safer benzodiazepines. Using alcohol as a sedative is not indicated. It causes very disrupted, nonrestful sleep as well as early-morning awakening and depression.

Any sedative should be used only as needed and on a limited basis if possible. Learning other techniques for relaxation as well as good sleep hygiene is always indicated. This includes such things as going to bed and awakening on a consistent schedule, no napping during the day, not doing anything stressful in bed, such as paying bills, and getting up if you don't fall asleep after thirty minutes and trying again when you feel more tired.

QUESTIONS TO ASK ABOUT MEDICINES

It is important to obtain accurate information about the medicine you are being prescribed for your back-pain problem. You should know the answers to the following questions before taking medications:

- Why am I being given this medication?

- What benefit should I expect and how long will it take to achieve?

- How should I take this medication (e.g., morning, night, with meals, on an empty stomach, every day, as needed)?

- What side effects should I be aware of? Will these go away?

- Can I take this medicine in addition to other medications I am on?

- How do I stop this medication safely?

SUMMARY

It is important to note that almost all of the medications we have mentioned for use in back pain have a large list of side effects, according to the *Physicians' Desk Reference* (PDR) and other books on drugs and medications. Patients often become extremely fearful of these side effects, as the lists can be quite overwhelming. Although we do not encourage the use of medications when it can be avoided, they are often very helpful and commonly used. We have seen that indiscriminate use of medicines does occur in medical practice and therefore it is important for the patient to be informed. It is important to discuss medication issues openly with your doctor.

Overall there is often a role for medications in chronic back-pain patients when properly selected by a physician knowledgeable in their use. Most medications, including anti-inflammatories, analgesics, muscle relaxants, antianxiety medication, and occasionally sedatives, should be limited to the acute periods if needed at all. With some medications (most notably the antidepressants) there is often a role for more long-term use. None of these medications should serve as a substitute for employing other important techniques in the individual's healing as discussed throughout this book.

CHAPTER 12

SPINE SURGERY: ALMOST ALWAYS A CHOICE

One would expect that the recommendation for a patient to undergo spine surgery would be a fairly straightforward process based primarily on medical need. One might also expect that spine surgeons generally agree upon which conditions are appropriate for surgery and which ones are not. In reality nothing could be farther from the truth.

As we shall see, there are almost as many definitions of "surgical need" as there are surgeons who perform such surgery. Factors that can affect surgical decision making include your symptom presentation, your diagnostic-test findings, how and where your surgeon was trained, how aggressive your surgeon is in terms of believing surgery is the answer, how much you want surgery, and your type of insurance. The most important message of this chapter is:

Spine surgery is almost always elective.

In some rare cases there may be an emergent need for spine surgery and serious consequences will occur if it is delayed. Generally these fall into three categories: cauda equina syndrome, tumors, and infections. This group, however, represents a very small minority of surgical cases. In many instances surgeons may predict dire consequences if surgery is not performed when in fact the procedure falls into the elective category.

This chapter will first discuss the three categories in which spine surgery may be a medical necessity. We will then give guidelines to help you understand the process of surgical decision making, followed by a review of the different conditions that are most commonly treated with elective spine surgery. Lastly we will present "red warning flags" related to spine-surgery practice. As each case is individual, this chapter will provide a general framework for you to use in working with your doctor.

MEDICALLY NECESSARY SPINE SURGERY

In the vast majority of cases we are able to tell the patient with back and/or leg pain that "This disorder won't kill you; it won't shorten your life or paralyze you; and the decision for spine surgery is absolutely elective." In rare cases there are spine disorders that may either be life-threatening or result in severe disability if surgery is not done. In general these include (a) a cauda equina syndrome; (b) a tumor in the spine; or (c) an infection in the spine in which there is rapidly progressive neurologic loss including bowel and bladder problems. These three conditions will be discussed in greater detail in the following sections.

Cauda Equina Syndrome

As discussed in the chapter on diagnosis, the telltale symptoms of a cauda equina syndrome may include genital numbness, numbness around the anus, loss of the feeling or urge that you have to urinate, inability to initiate urination, numbness in the feet, and loss of sexual function. If the condition is not surgically treated quickly, you may end up with permanent loss of bowel, bladder, and/or sexual function.

Although cauda equina syndrome is almost always caused by a herniated disc, having a disc herniation does not mean you are likely to get a cauda equina syndrome. Certain spine surgeons may mention this possibility without emphasizing its rarity in order to scare people into agreeing to have an elective spine surgery. We feel it is more appropriate to make patients aware of the associated symptoms of this condition and to instruct them to notify us immediately if they occur.

Tumors

If someone has a tumor involving the spine, surgery is frequently necessary, as a tumor tends to grow, albeit slowly. This is especially true in the thoracic and cervical areas, where the spinal cord may be involved. If you have a tumor in the lumbar spine where one nerve root is involved, a case could be made for watching it and allowing the person to live with the tumor if it is benign (noncancerous). In these cases there is no absolute indication for surgery except if the person has pain he or she cannot live with or significant loss of function. For surgery to be successful, the surgeon may have to "sacrifice," or destroy, the nerve involved in order to remove the lesion. Depending upon the particular nerve root, one can predict that there might be a loss of feeling or strength in the area of the body that the nerve controls, although precise outcomes can never be fully predicted.

Infection

The third area in which spine surgery might not be elective is that of infections in the spine. Just like other parts of your body, it is possible to get an infection in the spine. The length of time between the onset of infection in the spinal column and the time of diagnosis can be as long as six to twelve weeks. These patients are often misdiagnosed with what is initially believed to be a sprain or soft-tissue problem in the thoracic or lumbar area.

One "tip-off" symptom of a spine infection is pain at night. This is termed *rest pain* and involves a throbbing, aching pain that is worse with rest and can be quite severe. Although most people with a back-pain problem will report being awakened by the pain on occasion, this is different from the constant throbbing rest pain seen with infections. Infections can occur in either the disc space or the vertebral body, and these are basically separate conditions. Diagnosing an infection in the spine might ultimately include using imaging tests, bone scan, and blood tests.

How a person gets an infection in his or her spine is not completely understood. There are a few groups who might be predisposed to infection, among them those who have weakened immune systems (the "immunocompromised"). This can occur in such conditions as diabetes, chronic drug use, or someone on steroids (cortisone). If the person is immunocompromised and then undergoes a dental or genitourinary procedure, he or she can get germs in his or her bloodstream (bacteremia), which spread to the spine.

An infection in the spine is treated similar to other infections in the body, although there are some features that make it unique. First of all, the bacteria must be treated with IV (intravenous—"into the vein") rather than oral antibiotics. Surgical treatment may also be necessary to, in essence, clean out the area of the infection; however, most cases are successfully treated conservatively, without the surgical approach.

These three conditions represent the nonelective areas of spine surgery. The combined total of all cases that fit into these three areas probably account for no more than 1 percent of all the spine surgery done. *That makes approximately 99 percent of all spine surgery elective.*

ELECTIVE SPINE SURGERY

In the following sections we will discuss elective spine surgery, the most common site of which is the lumbar area. Overall, 1 to 3 percent of the population in the United States undergo a lumbar spine operation sometime during their lifetimes, and approximately 300,000 such operations are performed each year in this country. A majority of these surgeries are done to address one of three conditions: disc herniation/degeneration, spinal stenosis, and spondylolisthesis.

In this section we will discuss the following:

- Guidelines for surgical decision making to help you arrive at the best possible course of action

- Common problems treated with spine surgery

- How to find a good spine surgeon by gathering information, consulting a physical-medicine doctor, choosing between a neurosurgeon and an orthopedic surgeon, and finding a doctor who takes a human approach

- "Red flags" to be aware of in working with your surgeon

General Guidelines for Surgical Decision Making

Certain guidelines can be applied to almost any back-pain situation in which surgery is a possible treatment option. They will help you manage the situation more effectively and increase the probability of a positive outcome. The following issues should be considered in the surgical decision-making process:

- The issue of back pain versus leg pain needs to be effectively addressed and resolved. Surgery is very rarely appropriate for back pain when it is the only symptom. Most often, lumbar spine surgery is intended to treat leg pain (sciatica).

- Surgery should be considered if you are getting worse in the face of appropriate, aggressive conservative treatment. Failure of conservative treatment is an essential part of the decision for or against surgery.

- You may be finding your current symptoms absolutely unacceptable and you desire other options, such as the surgical approach.

- As a general rule, surgery should only be considered if your symptoms and physical/diagnostic test findings are consistent.

- You should be psychologically and emotionally equipped to manage the stress of surgery and postoperative rehabilitation as well as the possibility that the surgery will not work.

- There should be no factors (drug use, lawsuit issues, family issues, compensation, chronic pain syndrome, etc.) that would preclude you having a successful response to the surgery.

Each of these issues will be discussed in this chapter. These are important factors for you and your surgeon to consider in contemplating any elective spine surgery. They will help increase the chances of success following surgery to the highest possible level.

Leg Pain Versus Back Pain
The following statement is very important to remember when contemplating spine surgery:

Spine surgery for disc herniation in the lower back is virtually always to treat leg pain and/or buttock pain and not back pain.

Most low back problems that are appropriate for surgery include the symptom of pain down one or both legs. This is because the nerves that supply the legs pass through this area of the spine. This is also why a problem with the lower back (such as a disc herniation) will not necessarily be felt in the low back, and conversely low back pain is not necessarily associated with a structural problem in the lower spine. It is like having a telephone connection problem at the main switchboard that first shows up when there is static on your phone line at home. The problem is not in your home phone but rather at the main switchboard far away in another place. The problem must then be fixed at the switchboard and not in the home phone. Similarly leg pain is often a sign of a specific spinal problem, whereas back pain (by itself) is not.

Probably the most common reason for spine surgery is a disc herniation associated with pain in the low back, buttock, and going down one or both legs. One of the key issues in surgical decision making is to look at the natural history or healing process of a sciatica (leg pain) due to a disc herniation. The natural course of the problem is that 85 to 90 percent of the people can be treated effectively without surgery, although it may take up to twelve to sixteen weeks for the condition to heal. The healing process can be accelerated with effective ways of treating the acute radicular, or leg, part of the pain, which is caused by nerve-root inflammation. The nerve can get swollen when it's irritated from the piece of disc material that is either touching it or is in proximity to it. Because the herniated portion of the disc is mostly water, the piece that is causing the problem will tend to shrink with time. As the disc heals and shrinks, the irritation or pressure on the nerve is relieved. This is why most people get better without surgery.

There may be some rare instances when surgery for a disc problem is recommended for primary back pain, although, as we have discussed, the vast majority should be for leg pain. These instances include identification of a mechanical instability in the spine (spondylolisthesis) that is associated with mechanical-type back pain (pain that is alleviated with rest). If the pain can be reduced by having the patient wear a brace, resting, and by teaching him or her the appropriate stability exercises, then surgery can still be avoided. But if the symptoms of the instability do not resolve to a level that is acceptable to the patient, then a spine fusion can be considered.

Failure of Conservative Treatment
Another consideration in the question of surgery for back and leg pain is the effectiveness of aggressive conservative physical therapy. We must recognize that *conservative care is always an option.* One reason to consider a surgical approach is when there has been a failed conservative management attempt and there is still a degree of pain and disability. Even at this stage the decision to operate is still elective. This will depend on the physical findings as well as on the patient's needs. Typically if

someone has a herniated disc with sciatic pain and/or weakness in his or her lower extremity, a physical-therapy approach along with allowing the condition time to heal can be very effective.

When discussing conservative care it is very important to decide what constitutes a good trial of treatment. As we saw in chapter 8, many commonly used modalities are not effective. When we talk about an adequate course of conservative treatment, we mean that it includes such things as a specific active physical-therapy program, including spine-stabilizing exercises. The program will also often include learning proper body mechanics and how temporarily to avoid movements that are likely to aggravate the pain.

Surgery is still elective even after someone has "failed" conservative care. This is illustrated in the following scenario, which we see commonly: A surgeon will see someone with a disc herniation and nerve-root irritation causing sciatic pain. The first course of action will be some type of conservative care. If the patient fails the conservative care, the surgeon will then say, "Okay, that didn't work. It's time to try surgery." This is not a prudent course of action in many cases. It does not necessarily follow that a failed course of conservative therapy is an indication for surgery in and of itself. Surgery continues to be an elective decision. Whether or not a surgeon agrees with this view will depend greatly on how he or she was trained.

The Patient's Inability or Refusal to Accept the Symptoms
We would first begin considering the surgery option when the patient's symptoms are worsening in the face of appropriate aggressive conservative management and he or she finds the symptoms unacceptable. It is important to remember that

> **It is not whether the doctor finds the symptoms unacceptable but rather whether the patient finds them unacceptable.**

This is a very important differentiation because many spine surgeons try to dictate to the patient when to have surgery. In truth this decision is always the patient's.

You must be careful in assessing whether your symptoms are unacceptable and whether or not the conservative approach is working. People will often get impatient with the conservative treatment and be drawn to the "quick fix" idea of surgery. Thus another rule that we follow in surgical decision making is the following:

The patient who is improving should generally not consider the surgery option.

Discuss this issue with your doctor and physical therapist to help give you an accurate assessment of whether you are getting better. If you are, we believe you should allow yourself the possibility of continued improvement.

Even if your recovery is not complete and you do not regain 100 percent of your previous functioning, you don't have to have surgery if you are willing to live with your situation by altering your lifestyle somewhat, giving up certain activities to remain comfortable; and living with a certain amount of pain or discomfort while taking a minimum of pain medicines. If these trade-offs are ones the person finds acceptable, then surgery should not be done. We have had patients who have felt their situation was acceptable after conservative care even with some numbness, pain, and weakness. They basically made the decision "I'm okay with these symptoms and how they affect my life." The desired result of any treatment is that you, the patient, be satisfied.

Many spine surgeons will try to impose their own criterion for success upon you. This might include recommending surgery for a patient who is actually satisfied with residual symptoms after conservative treatment. Deciding against surgery at this point is perfectly acceptable, especially taking into account that surgery will very often not completely cure all the symptoms and can possibly make the problem worse.

Alternatively there is the person who is no longer getting better *and* finds his or her current symptoms unacceptable. In most of these cases the patient is not improving or is getting worse even after full involvement in the recommended conservative treatment for eight to twelve weeks since symptom onset. At this point in time you could talk about the appropriateness of surgery.

Consistency of Symptoms with Test Findings
It seems like an obvious statement that the patient's symptoms should be consistent with the test findings, but it is often violated by many surgeons anxious to provide the back-pain sufferer with a "cure." It is extremely important that the history and physical-examination findings be consistent with the diagnostic test results. Although this will be discussed extensively under the following sections, we will briefly address the issue here. For instance a person who has sciatica (leg pain) due to a disc herniation should have pain in a very specific area of the buttock and leg *that corresponds to the imaging studies and other diagnostic test results.* In other words the reason for the pain and other symptoms (numbness, weakness, etc.) must be able to be clearly established. When this is the case, surgery is highly successful.

Another scenario is unfortunately all too common. This is the patient who has not responded adequately to conservative treatment and has either minimal or inconsistent findings on the diagnostic tests and physical examination. For instance the patient might have minor findings on the MRI of disc bulging at one level but the pain in the back and leg does not match the disc problem. Thus it is unlikely that the disc bulges that were found are causing the pain problem. They may have been there for quite some time, not causing any symptoms at all. This case is not a surgical candidate regardless of the failure of conservative care. Yet a surgeon might be inclined to "give it a try" since nothing seems to be working. This "give it a try" attitude is rarely justified on the basis of the MRI findings when they do not match the physical-examination results. These surgeries are unlikely to be successful and may make the patient worse.

Psychological and Emotional Readiness of the Patient to Manage the Stress of Surgery and Rehabilitation
This issue will be fully addressed in chapters 14 and 15, but we will briefly summarize it here relative to spine surgery. Many surgeons will make surgical decisions based solely on the physical presentation without taking the whole person into account. They will do a physical and take a history, obtain the MRI and other diagnostic test results, conclude that the person is a surgical candidate, and schedule the surgery. This is what we call practicing "veterinary medicine" because the doctor does not listen to what the person is saying and feeling about his or her back problem.

There are several issues that may not make a person a good surgical candidate from an emotional standpoint. If this is the case, then some preparation for surgery from an emotional perspective is indicated. These issues might include the following:

- Depression

- Anxiety

- No support from family members or significant stress in family relationships

- Fear of the pain or previous negative experience with surgery

- Unrealistic expectations about surgery

- Other emotional or psychological concerns

If these issues are present, they should be addressed prior to surgery. Undergoing back surgery is a stressful medical procedure that can exacerbate such psychological and emotional issues. Many people (including spine surgeons) make the mistake of reasoning that "the surgery will fix the problem and

211

then you will have nothing to be upset about." However, there are many things that influence pain. If these other emotional factors are present, simply "fixing" the abnormalities in the spine will not solve the problem. We feel very strongly that

> **If these emotional issues are not addressed, the surgery can be a technical success but a clinical failure.**

The power of these emotional and psychological factors is only just now beginning to be understood. A recent study demonstrated how childhood psychological trauma influenced spine-surgery outcome. The study looked at eighty-six patients who underwent spine surgery and had between zero and five psychological risk factors experienced as a child, including (a) physical abuse; (b) sexual abuse; (c) alcohol or drug abuse in a primary caregiver; (d) abandonment; and (e) emotional neglect or abuse. Outcome from the surgery was assessed by looking at such things as whether repeat surgery was necessary, MRI of the spine six months after surgery, continued use of pain medicine more than six months after surgery, and ability or failure to return to work. The following table summarizes the results:

Number of Risk Factors	Probability of Successful Outcome from Surgery
0	95%
1	75%
2	43%
3	20%
4	7%
5	0%

As can be seen, the more risk factors, the less likelihood of a successful outcome from lumbar spine surgery. It is dramatic that even the presence of two risk factors decreases the success rate from 95 to 43 percent. The authors of the study concluded, "These reports support our observations that continued pain after technically successful lumbar spine surgery can in part be due to the psychological impact of severe childhood psychological trauma."

As of yet there is no good explanation for these findings, but they must certainly be taken into account in addressing the spine-surgery issue. Of course these data do not suggest that people with a history of abuse should never undergo spine surgery. They do suggest that if it appears this is an issue, psychological preparation for surgery or a psychological "screening" before surgery is indicated.

The Absence of Factors that Would Preclude a Successful Response to Surgery

Beyond the physical-examination findings, diagnostic test results, failure of conservative treatments, inability to accept the symptoms, and psychological factors, other issues can also impact the decision to recommend surgery and the outcome. They include such things as the following:

- Compensation/litigation issues

- Drug use

- The chronic pain syndrome

Ongoing compensation and/or litigation related to a spine problem is always of concern to us. These factors can affect the patient without him or her even being aware of it. Patients who are actively engaged in litigation or are on compensation related to their back pain are at risk for failed surgery. We have seen this time and again in the clinical setting and it has been established in the research literature. This is not to say that anyone involved in litigation is not a surgical candidate. Rather it is just one risk factor that requires presurgical assessment.

Our system of personal injury (at least in California) often reinforces continued disability and increased health care utilization. For instance in personal injury the amount of the lawsuit and settlement is often considered to be three times the amount of the total medical expenses. Of course with this as a guideline there can be subtle pressure to get the medical expenses as high as possible. There is no better (or quicker) way to do this than by having surgery. In some cases the attorney may be fairly straightforward about this issue, while in other cases the pressure is more subtle. The following case example illustrates this point:

Mr. B. was a forty-four-year-old man injured on the job while working as a postal carrier. He had back and leg pain due to a herniated disc at L4–5 (between the fourth and fifth lumbar vertebrae). Mr. B. responded well to an aggressive conservative therapy approach. He did have some residual pain and occasional numbness, but he was able to return to light-duty work and to resume most normal activities. He was in turmoil as to whether to consider the surgery option or to continue with more therapy. This was a highly litigated case including a workers' compensation claim and a personal injury claim. The treatment team decided to contact the patient's attorney (with permission) to try to get a feel for his attitude toward the patient and his improvement. The attorney basically stated that he did not care what kind of treatment the patient received as long as "at the final assessment the patient was rated as not being able to lift more than a pencil" (direct quote). This suggested that the attorney was communicating a similar strategy to the patient. We did not offer surgery to this patient under these conditions and encouraged continuing the conservative approach. The clear message from the attorney was that the more disabled the patient was at the time of settlement, the more the case would be worth.

Drug and alcohol use is another factor to be considered in the surgical decision-making process. If pain medication or other drug use is high, the patient may be at more risk for a poor surgical outcome. This is especially true if we believe the pain behavior and disability are being used in part as an excuse to take the pain medicines. Patients will also take pain medicines to medicate other nonphysical problems, such as depression and anxiety. The drug-use issue would have to be treated first and then the patient would be reassessed for the surgery option at a later time.

Lastly the more elements of the chronic pain syndrome that are present, the less likely a patient will respond positively to surgery. As discussed in other chapters, the chronic pain syndrome includes such things as pain that is inconsistent with physical findings, depression, anxiety, medication overuse, extended disability, sleep disruption, relationship problems, and so on. In these cases all the elements of the chronic pain syndrome must be treated simultaneously. Then if the patient responds adequately, the surgery option can be reassessed. Simply going in and "fixing" a structural spine problem without treating these other issues will, in virtually all cases, result in a failed-back-surgery case. Of course this will make everything even worse.

Common Problems Treated with Spine Surgery

Disc Problems

When discussing how to reduce leg pain (sciatic pain/nerve-root pain) due to disc problems, there are several factors that make a person a good surgical candidate. These include a person who has had an adequate trial of conservative treatment (e.g., the right kind of physical therapy, aerobics, anti-inflammatory medications, and possibly an epidural block or two) and who has pain that is consistent with the physical findings. As you will recall from chapter 5, nerves from the spine to the lower parts of the body serve specific areas. Sciatic-nerve problems will usually include pain in one leg along the "nerve-root distribution" and will most commonly present as pain below the knee. In addition we will look for other corroborative physical findings, such as

- A reduced ankle-jerk reflex, implying that there is a problem with the first sacral nerve root (L5–S1 disc)

- A reduced knee-jerk reflex, which would mean that there is a problem with the L4 nerve root (L3–L4 disc)

- A weak great-toe extensor tendon, which would imply a problem with the L5 nerve root (L4–L5 disc)

- A positive sciatic tension sign, as discussed in chapter 6.

If the patient demonstrates these symptoms, and an MRI or other imaging study shows a disc herniation consistent with the symptoms, surgery will most likely be successful—up to 94 percent of the time. However, before resorting to surgery, patients should first attempt a trial of aggressive physical therapy. Then if you have had the proper conservative treatment, are no longer improving, are in the eighth to sixteenth week from the onset of leg pain (not back pain), and find your symptoms unacceptable, surgery can be considered.

Even with all of these indicators you should keep in mind that sciatica often improves without surgery, as we discussed earlier. A study done by Dr. Henrik Weber in 1982 supports this claim. Dr. Weber compared a randomly assigned group of sixty-six patients who had surgery for sciatica due to a lumbar disc herniation with sixty patients who received conservative treatment. All of the patients had documented lumbar disc herniations with sciatic pain. The study assessed each group at one year, five years, and ten years after the treatment. Although the quality of life was slightly better in the first year in the surgical group, in the following nine years both groups showed similar improvements in all areas. Dr. Weber states, "In the nonoperated group 25% of the patients were cured (good) and 36% showed satisfactory improvement (fair). This means that approximately 60% of the operated patients may have been submitted to an unnecessary procedure." Clearly surgery is not the only cure for sciatica.

In addition to Dr. Weber's research, many studies using CT scans and MRIs have found that disc herniations can resolve either spontaneously or with conservative treatment. The results of Dr. Weber's study, and others, conclude that

> **The vast majority of disc bulge/herniations can be treated with a conservative approach and will not require surgery.**

Spinal Stenosis

As revealed in chapter 6, spinal stenosis is a narrowing of the spinal canal through which the neurologic/nerve elements pass. The narrowing is caused by bulging discs that are "worn out." In addition bone spurs from arthritis and a thickening of the ligaments of the spine can tend to make the spinal canal even smaller.

Stenosis results in a partial blockage of the blood flowing in the veins supplying the spinal nerves. When the person stands up and/or walks, it produces even further narrowing due to the shape of the spine (lordosis), causing a sensation of heaviness in the lower extremities and a feeling as if he or she can't walk. Sometimes the sensation is pain or numbness, but usually it is described as "I just can't walk as far; I get tired—my legs feel heavy."

There are two kinds of spinal stenosis. In *developmental* spinal stenosis the person is born with a smaller canal, and in *acquired* spinal stenosis it is due to degenerative changes that primarily occur in the elderly population. Most cases of stenosis are degenerative. One can also have a combination of the above, including aging/degenerative changes and a naturally small canal. For instance spinal stenosis that is symptomatic in a fifty-year-old is usually with a person who started out life with a small canal and it got too small by the time he or she was fifty, whereas a person with a normal-size canal may live to be eighty and not have difficulty.

This is a slowly progressive disease and only presents an emergency if there is a superimposed disc herniation in a person who has a very narrow spinal canal due to spinal stenosis. In this case one can have a sudden deterioration in neurologic function, such as a cauda equina syndrome, though the problem is very rare. The average patient has symptoms for months to years that slowly progress and he or she learns to adapt to them.

The conservative treatment for spinal stenosis is outlined in chapter 6. The indications for surgery for spinal stenosis are essentially the same as with sciatica due to a disc herniation, with one important exception. Unfortunately in spinal stenosis the natural history of the illness is not toward improvement but generally toward a worsening of the symptoms, because this is a degenerative disease. The conservative approach can be helpful in slowing down or stabilizing the symptoms, but usually will not eliminate them.

It should be kept in mind that surgery for spinal stenosis is elective and depends upon the patient's needs and response to conservative therapy. *Elective* is a very relative term. For an independent older woman who finds that she can't go shopping or take care of herself because she can't walk, or for someone who has retired recently and can't go on any trips because of the pain, it becomes important enough that he or she is willing to go through a moderately extensive spine surgery to address the problem. In these situations the patient may not feel the decision is really "elective" given his or her poor quality of life. On the other hand there are those people who basically have a very sedentary lifestyle and are willing to live within their limitations. For them this surgery is not a viable option.

It is critical in this patient population that their symptoms correlate with their radiographic studies and that spinal stenosis is in fact causing their problems. It is not uncommon to see spinal stenosis on the imaging studies of an elderly person in addition to symptoms of pain in the hips bilaterally (on both sides) and in the buttock. In some cases it turns out that the patient has a bursitis of the hip and/or degenerative arthritis of the hip, in addition to the spinal stenosis. The patient may have a surgery for spinal stenosis based on the scan and then still have the same pain. This is due to an incorrect diagnosis of the source of the pain, which comes from the bursitis in the hip area.

It is also important to distinguish between the symptoms of spinal stenosis and those due to vascular problems. Some of the symptoms, such as inability to walk fast or to walk certain distances, are very similar. Vascular disease (or "arteriosclerotic peripheral vascular disease") is basically inadequate blood flow, or poor circulation, to the legs. You don't have enough blood supply to keep up with the needs of your muscles. In this condition, just as in spinal stenosis, when people walk, their legs frequently start to hurt. Thus the pain could be due either to poor circulation, to the nerves being compressed in the spinal canal, or to a combination of both, since up to 8 percent of people with spinal stenosis also have vascular disease. Most of the time if the symptoms are caused by spinal stenosis, they will subside only if the person sits down and not simply if he or she stops walking.

Spondylolisthesis
As discussed in chapter 6, spondylolisthesis is a large word that simply means a slipping of one back bone (vertebra) on another. There are several kinds of spondylolisthesis and the two most common have been discussed previously in chapter 6.

Conservative treatment is often successful, although if it is not, a spinal fusion surgery may be recommended. The patient can then expect to be able to go back to his usual activities if the fusion is successful and the rest of his spine is normal. We generally see no reason for restrictions of any kind once approximately one or two years have passed since the fusion. Spine fusion surgery is discussed in the next chapter.

Finding a Spine Surgeon
Finding a spine surgeon to evaluate your problem can be a frustrating, scary, and expensive process, but a vitally important one, as it will determine how your treatment is managed. We have developed some guidelines that can help with this process:

- Gather information about the surgeon from several sources

- Consider a consultation with a physical-medicine and rehabilitation doctor (physiatrist) first

- Consider a consultation with an orthopedist who understands the conservative approach to spinal problems

- Consider finding an orthopedist or neurosurgeon who specializes in spine surgery

- Consider where you live and where your doctor was trained, as it will influence the surgery decision

- Find a surgeon who takes a human approach in addition to being technically skilled

Gather Information About the Referral

Your family doctor or chiropractor will usually be your first source of information about finding a spine surgeon. If a surgeon is required, it is usually prudent to get two or three individuals to choose from. There are several other sources of information that can be tapped beyond the initial referral by your doctor. It can be useful to ask family members or friends if they have any experience with physicians/surgeons who have treated back pain. You can also check with local-hospital physician-referral services and universities in the area. A family doctor in a given area usually has an idea about how the different spine surgeons approach their patients. Gathering information of this nature can give you a feel for how the surgeon practices and generally what impression people have of his or her work.

Consider a Consultation with a Physical-Medicine Doctor

Prior to making a surgical decision we recommend you consider a consultation with a physiatrist if possible. As presented earlier, a physiatrist is a rehabilitation doctor who treats patients with physical disabilities due to a variety of factors, including back pain. There is a relatively small number of physiatrists in the United States, so finding one who treats back pain can be challenging. Although physiatrists do not do surgery, they can help you decide whether further conservative treatment might be valuable or if surgery should be considered.

Consider an Orthopedist Who Understands and Utilizes a Conservative Approach

If you can't find a physiatrist, look for an orthopedic surgeon who utilizes an aggressive conservative approach. Here we mention an orthopedic surgeon as opposed to a neurosurgeon because as a rule most neurosurgeons have less training in rehabilitation methods. It may even be difficult to find an orthopedic surgeon with a really good understanding of aggressive physical-therapy approaches. We frequently see patients who report that they were treated by an orthopedic surgeon who prescribed the initial conservative physical therapy that did not work and now they are ready for surgery. But when we evaluate the physical-therapy approach used it was primarily "hummer/shake and bake" treatment (see chapter 8) with light exercise. In our opinion this is *not* an adequate trial of physical therapy prior to considering surgical alternatives.

Consider an Orthopedist or Neurosurgeon Who Specializes in Spine Surgery

When obtaining a consultation regarding the possibility of spine surgery, it is important to consider the training of the surgeon. There are many neurosurgeons and orthopedic surgeons who have a generalist practice in which they perform a wide variety of surgical procedures on many different parts of the body. Therefore getting an orthopedic surgeon who did a great operation on your friend's broken leg may not necessarily be your best resource for spine surgery. Finding a surgeon who either has a practice limited to spine surgery, has a great deal of experience in spine surgery, and/or has had fellowship training in spine surgery is probably the best course of action. If you live in a rural area, you may not have the luxury of these kinds of choices. Still, looking at the issue of training and experience may help you decide among the surgeons available to you in a specific area. Also if you have a particularly complex spine problem (such as a previous failed spine surgery), traveling to an academic institution or a center with physicians who specialize in spine treatment for a consultation will be very worthwhile.

There are often differences in how neurosurgeons and orthopedic surgeons approach spine problems. It is probably a safe assumption that in general neurosurgeons are more likely to recommend surgery for disc disease than orthopedic surgeons. Neurosurgeons as a group are less well trained in the rehabilitative treatment of spine disease, and thus they would be less likely to recommend it.

Another factor in deciding between a neurosurgeon and an orthopedic surgeon is whether or not a fusion is being considered. Fusions, in general, are not an integral part of the training of most neurosurgeons. If you are one of those people who need a spine fusion, you certainly should either have a consultation with an orthopedic surgeon in addition to a neurosurgeon or see a neurosurgeon with special training in the spine.

Consider Your Geographic Region

Location is another important factor to consider when looking for a spine surgeon. Surprisingly enough, the area of the country that a surgeon was trained in and/or practices in will influence the surgical decision-making process. Certain training programs are more in tune with the conservative management approach. If they have very strong rehabilitation and physical-therapy departments, and the professors in those departments are well versed in these issues, then that is what they are going to teach to their residents. If the surgeon you are seeing comes from a program where they are more inclined to think that everything is surgically correctable, then he or she will be more inclined to operate. Lastly the rate of back surgery can vary significantly between different countries and even within different regions of the United States.

Find a Surgeon Who Takes the Human Approach

Should you need the services of a spine surgeon, he or she should ideally be the kind of person with whom you feel you have a rapport and who is willing to educate you and answer your questions in a meaningful and appropriate way. Your surgeon should be someone who is not threatened by your questions. Your doctor should take the time to discuss different treatment options and other important issues with you.

Related to this issue, you must be very wary of the doctor who sees you as only a "spine" rather than as an entire human being. These types of surgeon are often simplistic in their clinical reasoning and appear to be more a technician than a complete physician. For a successful surgical result you should feel like you are working *with* your spine surgeon rather than being looked upon as a "bone spur" or "disc" to be removed.

"Red Flags" in Working with Your Spine Surgeon

The above-mentioned techniques will hopefully help you find a good spine surgeon. However, there are certain "red flags" to alert you to having found a "not so good" one. They are as follows:

- The surgeon basically allows no questions

- The surgeon does not encourage a second opinion or is threatened by your interest in one

- The surgeon suggests "exploratory" spine surgery

- The surgeon uses scare tactics

- The surgeon says, "I can cure you"

- The surgeon recommends surgery without a trial of conservative treatment (except in emergency situations)

Any of these warning signs is reason to run in the other direction as fast as you can without looking back. Each of these red flags will be discussed below.

The Surgeon Allows No Questions

One warning sign to watch out for is that your surgeon does not allow you to ask questions or treats the questions you ask with disdain. Of course if you go in with too many questions, you will lose your listener and not get the information you need. You can't expect the surgeon to answer pages and pages of questions. We recommend the following: Do not make the decision to have surgery on the first visit with the spine surgeon. The doctor should request that you come back again after you have had time to think about the options and to list your questions. If the doctor doesn't suggest the second visit, you should request it.

When you meet the doctor, you will get a sense as to whether he or she is the right kind of person for you. Does the doctor show compassion? Is he or she interested in educating you in the other methods of treatment, the risk/benefit ratio, the possible complications, and the reason for choosing that particular kind of surgery? These are all important issues. We strongly recommend getting answers to the following types of questions:

- What is my diagnosis and what does it mean to me?

- What is its natural course if left untreated?

- What are the treatment options?

- Why are you recommending a specific course of treatment?

- What are the risks and the benefits of each option?

If surgery is decided upon, then the following questions should also be asked and hopefully answered:

- What will the surgery entail?

- What are the possible complications and how are they treated?

- How will I feel after the surgery?

- How long will I be in the hospital?

- What will my recovery and rehabilitation be like?

- What preparations should I make to ensure the surgery is as successful as possible?

You have to beware of the doctor who says, "Don't ask questions. I'm the doctor. You'll do what I tell you." This is a significant red flag and suggests problems with the surgeon that will almost always negatively impact your treatment and eventual outcome.

The Surgeon Does Not Allow a Second Opinion or Is Threatened by It

We feel that prior to having surgery, it is appropriate either to get a second opinion or at least to ask the doctor who is recommending surgery how he or she feels about second opinions. If the doctor seems threatened by that question, *then you need a new doctor*. In our opinion any competent surgeon should welcome the opportunity of having a second opinion. Although your surgeon might not specifically recommend it, he or she should certainly agree that if you feel more comfortable having a second opinion, then you should definitely get it. In arranging for further consultation, it would be best to have two or three names from which to choose.

The Surgeon Suggests "Exploratory" Spine Surgery

There should be no such thing as "exploratory spine surgery." If any doctor says, "We are going to open you up and find out what's wrong and we'll fix it," take your X rays and run out of the office. There is no longer a place for surgeons who operate and decide what to do at the time of surgery. Given the availability of present-day sophisticated imaging studies (MRI, CT, myelograms, etc.), you should not be in an operating room unless the surgeon, and hopefully you, know almost exactly where the problem is and how to correct it—for instance, which nerve is causing leg pain, where it is being compressed and what is compressing it, and how to remove that compression effectively. Those issues should be addressed by the doctor and explained to you before the surgery.

The Surgeon Uses Scare Tactics

Another red flag we commonly see is surgeons using scare tactics to influence the surgical decision-making process. People frequently come to us who say, "I was told I need this spine surgery and that I may be paralyzed if I don't get it right away." As mentioned previously, a lower back problem leading to paralysis (e.g., cauda equina syndrome) is extremely rare. The following true example illustrates this type of scare tactic: A fifty-six-year-old woman came to us for a second opinion about a proposed spine surgery. The patient had a spinal stenosis with only mild symptoms. Her neurosurgeon had told her that if she did not have the surgery almost immediately, she would probably "end up in a wheelchair watching herself urinate on the floor." Needless to say, this was not an accurate statement, and even if there was a pressing need for surgery, this was not an appropriate manner in which to present it. As might be expected, the patient was very upset over this feedback regarding her condition. Scare tactics are generally not this aggressive, but can occur frequently in subtle forms. If you sense your surgeon is using these types of tactics, you should get a second or even third opinion.

The Surgeon Says, "I Can Cure You"

Some surgeons will tell their patients that a proposed surgery "should" cure them. It is implied to the patient, either directly or indirectly, that the surgery will be a simple procedure and that "of course" it will work. Any surgeon who presents the surgical option in this way is not being realistic and is not giving you full informed consent.

We have seen many cases in which the surgeon had made statements to this effect and convinced the patient to have surgery only to have the procedure not be successful. Unfortunately the surgeon will then (in most cases) tell the patient that "yes, the surgery was a technical success and the pain you are having must be due to something else." This can be very frustrating to the patient. The surgeon will then tell the patient that he or she has nothing else to offer. In more extreme cases the surgeon will offer yet another surgery to try to "cure" the problem again.

Any surgeon using this approach is not operating in your best interests.

The Surgeon Does Not Investigate a Conservative Treatment
As we have discussed, conservative management of most spine problems is well supported by both research and clinical evidence. It is important for your surgeon to be familiar with these conservative approaches in order to give you the best care possible. Your surgeon should question you about previous attempts at conservative care to ensure that they were carried out in the appropriate fashion.

Using these guidelines for finding a doctor can help ensure that you get the highest quality care and protect yourself from injury due to the treatment. Since many researchers in the field believe that a great majority of chronic back pain is due to inappropriate treatment by doctors, using these guidelines and being active in your own treatment is essential.

CHAPTER 13

SO YOU ARE GOING TO HAVE SPINE SURGERY

Surgeons must keep in mind that they operate on people, not on diagnostic studies.

As discussed in the previous chapter, the vast majority of spine surgery is elective; it is therefore essential to use that chapter's guidelines in the surgical decision-making process. They will help protect you from receiving unnecessary surgery.

If spine surgery is being considered or a decision has been made in a prudent manner, you should understand what it will entail and what to expect. Information of this nature can help the procedure go more smoothly and aid in your recovery. This chapter is meant only for the reader who has read the previous chapter and is seriously considering the surgery option. We must make the following warning:

> **Do not read this chapter before reading the prior one!**

This chapter will discuss the most common types of spine surgery including a description of the surgery, indications for the procedure, and the risks and benefits of each.

CHYMOPAPAIN INJECTION OR CHEMONUCLEOSIS

Description

Chemonucleosis is a process whereby an enzyme is injected into the intervertebral disc in order to chemically dissolve some of it. It is done to treat disc herniations and related sciatica.

The procedure is done in an outpatient setting, such as a hospital, surgery center, or X-ray suite. It is crucial that the injection be done under local anesthesia so that if the needle touches a nerve, both the patient and the surgeon will be aware and the needle can be redirected. It is also critical that the patient be tested to make sure that he or she is not allergic to the chemical enzyme, chymopapain.

Indications

The indications for a chymopapain injection are sciatic pain due to disc herniation that has not been alleviated after six to eight weeks of appropriate conservative treatment. The symptoms should be correlated with an MRI or CT scan abnormality at the appropriate level, as well as with clinical evidence of nerve-root irritation. It is not indicated in a person with spinal stenosis or if a significant loss of strength in one or both lower extremities is seen.

Risks and Benefits

Chymopapain injections were approved by the FDA for use in the United States in 1982 and the procedure had a brief period of popularity in the United States in the mid 1980s. Because of associated unpredictable neurological complications and allergic reactions to the chymopapain, it fell out of favor. It is still used with frequency in Canada, as well as in many countries in Europe. The reported success rate is 65 to 80 percent for sciatica, in properly selected patients.

The risks for chymopapain injections are a disc space infection, an allergic reaction to the enzyme, and paralysis due to a reaction to the enzyme. Unfortunately the risk of paralysis cannot be predicted with certainty, and this is why the procedure is rarely done in the United States.

PERCUTANEOUS DISCECTOMY

Description
Percutaneous discectomy is the surgical removal of a portion of the disc using a laser or suction device. It is primarily used in cases of sciatica due to disc herniation. The procedure is typically done on an outpatient basis in a hospital operating room, surgery center, or X-ray suite.

As with chemonucleosis, the patient is awake in order to avoid nerve injury during placement of the probe into the disc. The surgeon is guided in proper placement of the probe by visualization with fluoroscopic X ray. Barring complications, the patient is usually up and about and able to return to sedentary-type work and limited activities within forty-eight to seventy-two hours following the procedure.

Indications
The indications for percutaneous discectomy are patients who have uncomplicated sciatic pain for a minimum of six weeks and preferably ten to twelve weeks. These patients should have attempted appropriate aggressive conservative management and have a corroborative MRI study or CT scan.

As mentioned above, this procedure is typically used in cases of sciatica due to disc herniation. It can also be appropriate in cases of intermittent severe attacks of low back pain associated with a sciatic scoliosis. This is a condition in which a disc herniation (usually at L4–5) causes severe spasming of muscles on one side of the spine resulting in scoliosis or a curvature of the spine to the side.

Risks and Benefits
The risks associated with percutaneous discectomy are rare and include disc space infection, nerve or blood vessel injury, or recurrent herniation. Recurrence of symptoms occurs in up

to 20 to 30 percent of patients within three to six months of the procedure.

This surgical procedure is currently being heavily advertised by doctors and hospitals. Despite reports of success in up to 80 percent of patients, in our experience this procedure actually has very limited usefulness for the treatment of sciatica. We believe the usefulness of percutaneous discectomy is quite limited, taking into account the success rate of conservative treatment and that those who fail conservative treatment seem usually to fall into a category of patients who do very well with a microsurgical discectomy.

MICROSURGICAL DISCECTOMY

Description
The operation is an "open" surgical procedure done with a microscope and requires a laminotomy (which will be discussed more fully later), or partial removal of a small amount of the lamina (this is the bone covering the spinal canal—see chapter 5). The patient is hospitalized the morning of the procedure, which is done under general anesthesia and can take anywhere from forty-five minutes to several hours depending on what has to be done. The procedure generally requires a very small incision (1 to 1½ inches).

Indications
Microsurgical discectomy for a herniated disc is indicated for sciatic pain that is unrelieved after conservative treatment, progressive neurological loss causing significant problems in daily functioning, spinal stenosis in older patients associated with a disc herniation causing the sciatic pain, and recurrent disc herniations. In addition it is infrequently indicated in the older population with spinal stenosis and resultant inability to walk due either to pain or to a sense of weakness in the lower extremities, although this group of patients is usually treated with a laminectomy (to be discussed elsewhere in this chapter).

Recovery and Rehabilitation

The recovery period after surgery is usually twenty-four to forty-eight hours in the hospital, and most patients are walking by the morning following the surgery. The pain following this type of surgical procedure is minimal and is usually controlled with limited pain medicines. The majority of the local discomfort from the surgery subsides within several days; however, the sciatic pain may take up to eight weeks to subside completely.

We suggest to our patients that they remain at home for approximately one week following discharge from the hospital. They are allowed to walk about, sit, stand, or lie down as their comfort allows. Driving short distances is usually permitted at about seven to ten days following surgery, and return to sedentary and semisedentary types of occupations is allowed, at least on a part-time basis, usually within about the same time period.

Risks and Benefits

The risks of the microsurgical discectomy include infection, injury to the nerve root, problems with the anesthesia, a blood clot, and recurrent disc herniation. In order to prevent infection, an antibiotic is given intravenously (into a blood vessel) at the time of surgery and occasionally eight hours following the surgery. Necessary nerve-root manipulation during surgery can result in injury causing numbness and/or weakness in the distribution of the involved nerve. These symptoms often resolve over a period of several months after surgery.

Problems with anesthesia are very rare, as is the possibility of a blood clot forming in the legs. In an attempt to prevent this latter complication, support stockings are used during the surgery and after, until the patient is up and walking.

There is approximately a 4 percent chance of a recurrent herniation of additional disc material at the operated level. This is due to the fact that no attempt is made at the time of surgery to remove the entire disc, but rather only that portion that is causing the compression/irritation of the nerve root. Thus there is always the rare possibility of some of the remaining disc material herniating. Although we make every attempt to remove that portion of the disc that is obviously degenerated, approximately 60 to 70 percent of the nucleus pulposus or soft portion of the disc is left intact. For whatever reasons that caused the initial disc herniation, additional degeneration can take place and another piece of disc can work its way out through the opening of the cover (annulus) and cause a reherniation and recurrent sciatic pain.

If reherniation occurs, there will usually have been a pain-free interval following a successful microsurgical discectomy with a sudden recurrence of sciatic pain. This recurrence in pain is almost always due to a recurrent disc fragment, and often the pain is much more intense than the initial sciatica. This is because scarring around the affected nerve from the initial surgery causes the nerve to be less able to "move away" from the irritating fragment of disc. In these situations the use of oral steroids for a period of five to seven days and/or one or two epidural blocks will sometimes successfully treat the problem (about 30 to 40 percent of the time). Because of the severe pain often associated with reherniation, doing repeat surgery fairly quickly is required in the remaining patients (about 60 to 70 percent), and it is usually quite successful.

LAMINOTOMY AND FORAMINOTOMY

Description
A laminotomy involves creating a limited opening through the lamina allowing access to the spinal canal. A foraminotomy involves making a larger opening in the intervertebral foramina to relieve nerve-root compression. The foramina is a natural opening (e.g., "hole") in the spinal canal that allows the nerve root to emerge and join with other nerves to form the sciatic nerve, which passes out of the spine into the buttock and down the leg to the lower calf (see figure 5-8).

Indications
A laminotomy in essence is what is done during the course of a microsurgical discectomy. In older people who have sciatica

due to a disc bulge (without herniation) and a limited opening for the emerging nerve due to "bone spurs," or calcium deposits, a foraminotomy is also done. This simply means removing additional bone with a high-speed drill laminotomy. These procedures result in more room for the nerves, which in turn takes care of the pressure causing irritation.

Risks, Benefits, and Recovery
The preoperative evaluation, the length of surgery, the complications, and the usual postoperative course of events are the same for laminotomy/foraminotomy as they are for microsurgical discectomy.

LAMINECTOMY

Description
A laminectomy is the surgical removal of the lamina and associated ligament in order to get to a herniated disc, which is then removed, alleviating the pressure and irritation of the affected nerve root or roots. A laminectomy is also done to decompress (take the pressure off) the canal in cases of spinal stenosis. The patient is admitted to the hospital the morning of the surgery and stays between two to five days, depending upon the person's age and overall functioning.

Indications
The indications for a laminectomy are a large disc herniation causing a cauda equina syndrome and/or conditions associated with advanced spinal stenosis. A laminectomy can also be an appropriate treatment for those people who may have had prior surgery with recurrent and/or residual problems requiring additional bone removal and a full decompression of the nerves.

Recovery and Rehabilitation
Although the hospital stay is typically two to five days, in the elderly population (seventy to ninety years old) it is often nec-

essary to have additional rehabilitation in an extended-care facility for a period up to several weeks. Because a laminectomy is done primarily in conditions of spinal stenosis, the recovery period and the resolution of symptoms is longer than it would be following surgery for acute sciatic conditions due to a simple disc herniation. We advise our patients that recovery can take up to four to six months and sometimes even longer. This is especially true in regard to the patient's ability to walk reasonable distances. Postoperative rehabilitation often requires physical therapy started within two to three weeks of the operation and continuing for up to four to six weeks.

Risks and Benefits

In a full laminectomy the risk of infection or of a blood clot is somewhat greater than in the microsurgical procedures, due to the longer operating time. The risk of disc reherniation and need for reoperation after a laminectomy is between 4 and 6 percent.

SPINAL FUSION

Description

A fusion is an operation wherein the surgeon attempts to stop the motion that normally takes place between two adjacent vertebral bodies. There are basically two types of fusions: the posterior approach and the anterior approach. Sometimes a spinal fusion may involve the use of instrumentation ("metal rods").

The vast majority of fusions are done from the posterior, or back, approach. Initially the outer hard-bone portion of the transverse processes is removed. As discussed in chapter 5, the transverse processes are the portions of the vertebral body that stick out to the side. Fresh bone is then taken from the patient's iliac crest (the hip) and laid on the transverse processes, with the goal that eventually they will grow together. This is called a lateral or transverse-process fusion and is the most common type done. Once the bone grows together, the two vertebrae form one solid unit with almost no motion between them.

The second type of fusion is called an anterior fusion because it is done from the front of the spine. It requires an incision in the abdominal or flank area in order to access the front of the spine. Due to the complexity of this procedure, it is our opinion that there should be both a spine surgeon and either a general surgeon or a vascular surgeon whenever possible. This team of different surgical specialists will increase the safety of the surgery. This type of fusion also usually requires removal of several portions of bone from the patient's hip to be inserted between the two vertebral bodies. This is done after the disc has been removed and the two vertebral bodies have been properly "prepared" so that the bone graft will grow.

Indications

Spinal fusion is indicated much less frequently than any of the procedures previously discussed. The primary indication is for alleviation of "mechanical" low back pain. This is pain that is made worse by activity such as bending, twisting, and lifting, and improved by rest, usually in a recumbent position. For a fusion to be successful, one should have a "worn out" or degenerative disc between the two adjacent vertebral bodies in question and preferably some form of abnormal motion or instability between the vertebrae involved. This instability can be increased by bending forward or backward, or by an actual slipping of one bone on the bone below (see spondylolisthesis). These abnormal motions can sometimes be demonstrated on "bending" X-ray films, in which the patient bends forward and backward while X rays are taken and evaluated in both positions.

Fusion surgery is *not* indicated for the treatment of leg pain, except in very rare instances. Neither should it be considered for those individuals who have back pain that appears to be on the basis of muscular and/or ligamentous strain and is not associated with an identifiable mechanical abnormality involving the vertebral bodies, the associated discs, and/or the joints.

Spinal Fusion with Instrumentation

During the past several years there has been a significant increase in the use of instrumentation in spinal fusions. This involves the use of such things as pedicle screws (screws that are anchored into the pedicles; see chapter 5) as well as plates and rods that connect the screws together. This instrumentation is felt to improve the chances of obtaining a successful fusion.

Since attempting to fuse more than one level lowers the chances of obtaining a successful fusion, many surgeons feel that this type of instrumentation should be considered in these cases. It should be noted that the definition of a "successful fusion" is that it is solid (the bones grow together). This should not be confused with the success of the surgery overall in terms of relieving the patient's symptoms. Another indication for the use of pedicle screws is in smokers. People who smoke have been shown experimentally to have significantly less chance of obtaining a successful fusion (as low as 60 percent compared with 85 percent in the nonsmoking population). Instrumentation may also be indicated in patients who have had a prior attempted fusion that has failed and in people with significant instability.

In rare instances it is appropriate to do a posterior and an anterior fusion. This might be necessary for people who have had failed prior surgeries, who are smokers, and/or who have had prior complications such as infection. In these cases two separate surgical procedures are done, either under a single anesthetic or several days apart.

Recovery and Rehabilitation

The recovery period following a fusion operation is understandably longer and is associated with a significant degree of postoperative pain compared with other spine surgeries. Patients are often hospitalized for a period of up to one week. It is unusual for a patient to be able to return to even sedentary work in less than two to three weeks.

For either an anterior or a posterior fusion it is almost always necessary for the patient to wear a brace for a period of three to four months following the surgery. The brace is often made out of a custom-fitted lightweight plastic and can be worn under the patient's clothes. In many instances it can be removed when the patient is in bed. The use of such a bracing device, even when pedicle-screw instrumentation is in place, is felt to improve the chances of obtaining a solid fusion by as much as 5 to 10 percent.

Rehabilitation following a spinal fusion usually does not begin until several months after the surgery. During that initial two-month phase the patient is encouraged to walk either outside or on a treadmill, and occasionally will be allowed to use an exercise bicycle. Formal physical therapy is recommended to begin approximately two to three months after surgery.

Risks and Benefits of Fusion Surgery

The risks associated with a spine fusion are significantly greater than those associated with a simple laminotomy and/or discectomy, although they are still quite low. Generally the risks are similar to those of previously discussed surgeries but at a higher rate. Other risks include a failure or breakage of the instrumentation, pain in the hip where the bone graft is taken from, infection, and failure of the vertebrae to fuse.

Given such things as the greater length of time off from work, the significant cost, and the longer rehabilitation time associated with this major surgery, consideration of the risk/benefit ratio should be done with great care. In our experience a fusion should *not* be done on a person with sciatica simply due to a disc herniation. In these cases it has been shown in numerous studies that the results from a simple laminotomy and discectomy are equal to or superior to those following a discectomy and fusion.

There have been several recent national news reports regarding complications associated with the use of pedicle screws, plates, and rods (the "instrumentation"). It has been asserted that certain types of these screws are prone to breaking and that the instrumentation is not currently fully approved by the Food and Drug Administration (FDA) for use in spine surgery. There have been, however, 50,000 to 70,000 such surgeries done in the United States yearly for the past several years. The issue of the type and manufacturer of the instrumentation as well as of FDA approval should be discussed fully with your surgeon if you have been recommended for such a surgery.

If a spinal fusion with instrumentation has been recommended for you, it is imperative that you obtain at least one second opinion from a qualified spine surgeon. In addition it is important that the surgery be performed by orthopedic surgeons or neurosurgeons who have had additional training and/or significant surgical experience doing these procedures and using these types of materials (the instrumentation). In our opinion the risks associated with the use of pedicle screws and instrumentation are greatly increased if attempted by the "occasional" spine surgeon. We cannot recommend strongly enough that surgery of this type be done by surgeons specializing in spine surgery.

PREPARING FOR SURGERY

Preparing for spine surgery can be divided into medical, psychological, and psychosocial aspects. It is important to consider all of these areas in order to help increase the probability of a successful outcome. Of these, most surgeons focus primarily on the medical aspects of the surgery to the exclusion of the other two areas, but these latter should be assessed and addressed as well. We will discuss these three areas of preparation in the following sections.

Medical Preparation for Surgery

Medical preparation for spine surgery can include several things. First, depending on the surgery being performed, a consultation with an internist may be required to ensure that the patient can safely undergo the procedure.

Second is a review of the medications the patient is taking. We generally have all of our patients stop taking aspirin, aspirin-containing compounds, nonsteroidal anti-inflammatories, and blood-thinning medications for a period of at least three to ten days prior to surgery, depending on the medicine. Patients on these compounds can have increased bleeding, which can lead to complications during or following the surgical procedure. Depending on the situation, the medication can be started again after surgery, as directed by your doctor.

Third, a patient who is smoking and is scheduled for spine fusion is required to stop smoking for a period of a minimum of four to six weeks prior to surgery. This is absolutely necessary in order to improve the chances of obtaining a successful fusion. As discussed previously, taking all other factors into account, the success rate for a fusion surgery is much less in smokers as compared with nonsmokers. The accepted explanation at this time for the significant increase in failure of fusion in smokers is that the nicotine causes constriction of the small blood vessels, which are necessary to bring blood to the area of the fusion. In a successful fusion the vertebral "bones" grow together, and for this to occur the area needs an adequate supply of new blood.

Psychological Preparation for Surgery

Psychological screening and preparation for surgery can be important, especially for those patients who have had prior unsuccessful surgeries and/or are having an extensive operation, such as a posterior laminectomy/fusion with or without instrumentation, or those few that are having anterior and posterior fusions. In these cases we feel it is crucial that the patient undergo a psychological evaluation preoperatively with a psychologist who is skilled in evaluation and management of chronic pain patients. This preoperative evaluation addresses such issues as have been discussed in the previous chapter.

In some cases a brief psychological preparation for surgery program might be instituted. This would include such things as giving the patient an opportunity to discuss any anxiety or fears, his or her expectations about the experience, and the predicted course of events. This preparation also includes making sure the patient has accurate information about what to expect before and after the hospital stay as well as relaxation training for more effective pain and anxiety control. Research has shown that this type of treatment can help decrease post-operative pain, decrease time in the hospital, decrease disability time after the operation, decrease the need for pain medicine, and improve the chances for a successful outcome overall.

In our opinion the rehabilitation of patients with complicated chronic spine problems requires a multidisciplinary approach including, but not limited to, evaluation by a physical-medicine and rehabilitation physician as well as an appropriate psychologist. Without such preoperative and postoperative guidance, the chances of obtaining a success result in this group of patients can be greatly diminished.

Psychosocial Preparation for Surgery

Psychosocial issues that might be addressed presurgically include such things as the work situation and the family. Prior to the microdiscectomy type of surgery it is generally unnecessary for the patient to stop working. We actually encourage a person to continue with his normal activities (including a normal exercise program, or whatever he is capable of) up until the time of the surgery. This is done to keep the patient as physically and emotionally healthy as possible. Unfortunately most of the patients requiring surgery are unable to perform any of these activities, and that is in fact the reason they are having the surgery.

In addition to encouraging patients to engage in normal activities until the time of surgery, we attempt to address any other problems. These might include such things as resolving insurance and financial issues, discussing when the patient might be able to return to work and helping him or her get this cleared with the employer, addressing when the patient can return to a more active lifestyle including exercise, and helping the family cope with the patient's postoperative rehabilitation period. Our institute believes that for a select group of patients it is necessary for these issues to be addressed for a successful postsurgical outcome.

POSTOPERATIVE REHABILITATION

Knowing what to expect as far as the postoperative recovery time, postoperative pain control, and rehabilitation is a key factor in having realistic expectations regarding surgery. Studies have shown that when patients are prepared for surgery by being given appropriate expectation of what to expect, they will do better and recover faster.

For pain control in the hospital after a spine surgery such as a full laminectomy for spinal stenosis or a laminectomy and fusion in the younger-aged patient, we are now using patient-controlled analgesia (PCA). In using this equipment the patient has an IV placed and he or she can simply press a button to get an appropriate dose of pain medicine directly into the bloodstream. This allows the patient to prevent the pain from becoming severe while reducing anxiety since he or she does not have to call for a nurse and wait to get the pain medicine. Research has shown that the use of PCAs results in less pain medicine being needed overall with much better pain control. PCAs can be associated with some significant side effects in the older population and thus are used less frequently in this group.

If a PCA is used following an extensive spine surgery, such as a full laminectomy and/or fusion, it is usually for twenty-four to forty-eight hours postoperatively. It is then supplanted by the use of either injectable narcotic medication or appropriate oral medication. Patients are discharged on oral pain medication, which is tapered as healing takes place and the pain subsides.

Most spine surgeries will require some type of physical therapy postoperatively. The timing and type of this treatment will vary depending upon the surgery completed. It is important that the patient have an understanding of when this will begin, what it will entail, and what exercise and activities can be done at home.

For the person undergoing an outpatient procedure (e.g., percutaneous discectomy) or a limited surgical procedure (e.g., microsurgical discectomy or foraminotomy), it is usually not necessary to make extensive arrangements for postoperative nursing care and so forth. These people are often started into a physical therapy program postoperatively for a brief period in order to reinforce the appropriate types of exercises and spine mechanics. This can help to prevent reinjury and to facilitate getting the patient to return to an active lifestyle as soon as is medically possible.

For the older individual it is crucial that arrangements be made for transition to the extended-care facility and eventually to the home environment. This issue should be addressed preoperatively in order to reduce any uncertainty or stress. In these instances home visits by a physical therapist, occupational therapist, and nurse may be appropriate for a brief time after discharge. Visits by a nurse are usually only necessary if there are wound problems. For the elderly individual with ambulatory problems entering the hospital for purposes of a laminectomy (usually for the treatment of spinal stenosis), it is imperative that the Social Services Department of the hospital be involved in the evaluation of the patient early on, and that arrangements be made for the patient to be transferred to the appropriate facility or to home with ancillary services. This helps greatly to reduce the patient's anxiety as well as the anxiety of those of the family members who are unable to "cope with" the patient's needs without this ancillary help.

PART IV

THE POWER
OF THE MIND
IN BACK PAIN

CHAPTER 14

BACK PAIN AND SUFFERING

Those who have something better to do, don't suffer as
much.   —*W. Fordyce, Ph.D.*

As we discussed earlier, there are many things that can increase or decrease your perception of pain. These influences
on pain perception are explained by the gate-control theory.
This chapter will be a further discussion of these issues, as it is
an area most commonly neglected in traditional approaches to
back pain. These factors are well known to the research and
academic communities but rarely acknowledged in general
practice.

YOUR PAIN SYSTEM

As we have discovered previously in discussing the gate-
control theory of pain, there is not a one-to-one relationship
between tissue damage and pain, as the specificity theory pos-
tulated. Rather, many factors influence back pain, disability,
and suffering. As we have stated many times throughout this
book, a person can have severe pain with minimal physical
findings and minimal pain with horrendous physical findings.
    The model pictured on page 248 describes, in a simple for-
mat, what is currently known about aspects of back pain. Although this may seem complicated at first, the model makes
common sense given the examples discussed in chapter 4,
such as hypnosis and phantom-limb pain. It may also be helpful
to think of personal experiences in which you had a minor

injury with severe pain or a major injury with little pain. These experiences are explained by the pain-system model.

The following are definitions of the various "layers" of pain in the model:

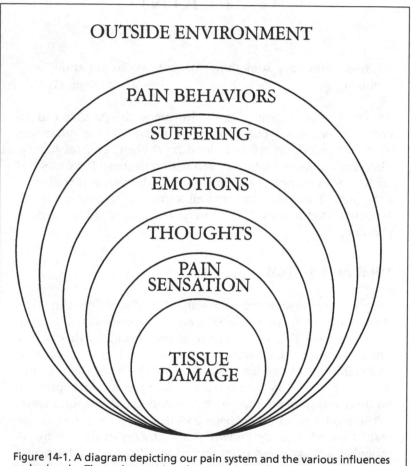

OUTSIDE ENVIRONMENT

PAIN BEHAVIORS

SUFFERING

EMOTIONS

THOUGHTS

PAIN
SENSATION

TISSUE
DAMAGE

Figure 14-1. A diagram depicting our pain system and the various influences on back pain. Tissue damage is only one of many factors determining how much pain will be experienced. Illustration provided courtesy of Century City Hospital, Los Angeles.

Tissue Damage, or Nociception

This is defined as mechanical, thermal (heat or cold), or chemical energy acting on specialized nerve endings that send an impulse, or "signal," into the nervous system that negative events are occurring. This is usually the beginning point of the "pain" message. It might include an impact or trauma (mechanical, such as cutting yourself), an injury involving temperature (thermal, such as burning yourself), or an injury involving chemical changes (chemical, such as an irritant). Nociception is what occurs at the site of injury that usually leads to pain being experienced. For instance, if you have ever hit your finger with a hammer or struck your toe on a table, you may have noticed that the pain signal can take a brief moment to reach your brain and be experienced.

Pain Sensation

This is the actual perception that occurs in the brain after the nerve signal travels from the periphery to the central nervous system. Pain sensation is experienced in the brain, while nociception occurs at the site of injury.

Thoughts

Cognitions or thoughts occur in higher brain centers and are an assessment of the pain-sensation signal coming into the nervous system as well as events surrounding it. These thoughts can be conscious or unconscious and will greatly influence how the pain signal is perceived. For instance general body aches and stiffness are perceived as "good pain" when these occur after a vigorous exercise session, whereas they are perceived as "bad pain" when related to a medical condition, such as fibromyalgia. The level of actual input to the nervous system may be the same, but the thoughts about the input cause the pain in the patient with fibromyalgia to be perceived as much more distressing.

Another example was experienced by Dr. Deardorff. As a teenager he was struck in the face by a door, causing a significant injury with profuse bleeding that required forty stitches. Interestingly *no* pain was experienced until the extent of the injury was realized by seeing the reaction of others and looking in the mirror. After that the pain became quite intense. These examples illustrate how thoughts (conscious and unconscious) impact pain perception and suffering. The thoughts were generally of the nature, "Oh . . . this must be very serious!" which made the pain worse.

In the case of back pain a similar assessment of the situation occurs in our unconscious. We have seen many patients who are convinced that their back pain represents serious damage even though physical findings are minimal. They believe that hurt equals harm and are totally guided and controlled by the pain. In these people suffering is very great. Alternatively we have seen people (a smaller group by far) who have very severe findings on their diagnostic test (e.g., MRI, CT) yet who don't seem to be bothered by the pain. They perceive their pain as benign or nondangerous. They live their lives regardless of the pain, and overall suffering is thereby diminished. Thus these differences in pain sensation can be explained by differences in thoughts and attitudes about the pain.

Emotions

The emotional aspect of your pain is your response to your thoughts about the pain. If you believe (thoughts) the pain is a serious threat, then emotional responses will include fear, depression, and anxiety, among others. Conversely if you believe the pain is not a threat, then the emotional response will be negligible. Consider, again, the previous example of a strenuous workout. The day afterward the person may show grimacing, slow movements, and other "pain behaviors." Even so, the thoughts about the pain will be positive ("Boy, what a good workout that was last night") and the emotions will follow similarly (e.g., feeling good about having worked so hard).

We will further discuss the emotional aspects of pain later in this chapter.

Suffering

Suffering is very closely tied to the emotional aspect of pain. In general it is triggered by aversive events, such as loss of a loved one, fear, or a threat to one's well-being. Suffering very often occurs in *anticipation* of a *possible* perceived threat even though the threat may or may not actually exist.

A very good example of this last scenario was presented in chapter 4. A patient with severe headaches was firmly convinced she had a brain tumor. Her husband had recently died of a brain tumor that had started with simple headaches. Her suffering was very high, since she was anticipating her headaches were a sign of a very serious condition that could lead to death. After the MRI it was confirmed that she did not have a tumor and that her headaches were likely due to muscle tension. Her suffering decreased significantly, as did her pain. This illustrates extreme suffering in response to a threat that never actually exists.

Pain Behaviors

Pain behaviors are defined as things people do when they suffer or are in pain. These are behaviors that others *observe* as typically indicating pain, such as grimacing, limping, taking pain medicine, moving slowly, and asking for help. Pain behaviors are in response to all the other factors in the pain-system model (tissue damage, pain sensation, thoughts, emotions, and suffering). Pain behaviors are also affected by previous life experiences, expectancies, and cultural influences in terms of *how* the pain is expressed. Interestingly pain behaviors are also affected by the outside environment, as will be discussed in the next section.

Psychosocial Environment

Psychosocial environment is a fancy term for the environments in which we live, work, and play. Research has consistently shown that these environments influence how much a person will show pain behaviors. Back pain can affect all aspects of a person's life including relationships, work activity, sexual functioning, recreational pursuits, and so on. Exactly how these environments can affect your pain and suffering will be discussed in great detail in later sections.

FACTORS INFLUENCING ACUTE AND CHRONIC PAIN

As we discussed in chapter 4, pain can be divided into acute and chronic phases based upon the length of time in pain and how fast the tissues are expected to heal. It is very important to understand that as pain moves from the acute to the chronic stages, the influences of other factors in the pain system (aside from tissue damage) come more into play. This is illustrated in the following model:

As can be seen in this model, as back pain goes on longer and longer, factors *other than tissue input* become more influential. This can be a difficult concept for patients to understand, and the common retort is, "But I have real pain." Again, as a reminder, the pain is absolutely real and is physically experienced. It is simply being supported and increased by factors other than the tissue damage. Remember, in these cases, *hurt does not equal harm or tissue damage!!*

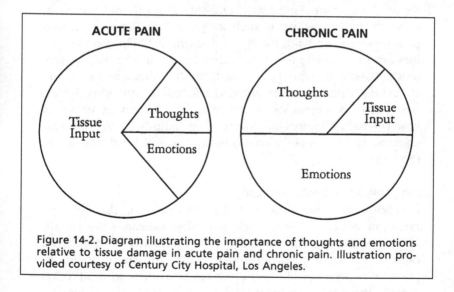

Figure 14-2. Diagram illustrating the importance of thoughts and emotions relative to tissue damage in acute pain and chronic pain. Illustration provided courtesy of Century City Hospital, Los Angeles.

PAIN AND EMOTIONS

As we discovered in the pain-system model, thoughts, emotions, and suffering are an integral part of any back-pain experience. In this section we will further investigate how emotions influence pain and vice versa. These emotions include depression, anxiety, fear, and anger.

Depression

Depression is placed first on the list, as it is by far the most common emotion associated with chronic back pain. The type of depression we are discussing goes beyond what would be considered normal sadness or feeling "down" for a few days. This depression (referred to as major or clinical depression) includes such symptoms as the following:

- A predominant mood that is depressed, sad, blue, hopeless, low, or irritable. This may include periodic crying spells

- Poor appetite or significant weight loss or increased appetite or weight gain

- Sleep problem of either too much or too little sleep

- Feeling agitated (restless) or sluggish (low energy or fatigue)

- Loss of interest or pleasure in usual activities; social isolation

- Decreased sex drive

- Feelings of worthlessness and/or guilt

- Problems with concentration or memory

- Thoughts of death, suicide, or wishing to be dead

Major depression is thought to be four times greater in people with chronic back pain than in the general population. In research studies on depression in chronic low-back-pain patients seeking treatment at pain clinics, prevalence rates are even higher. These range from 32 to 82 percent of patients showing some type of depressive problem, with an average of 62 percent.

Depression is more commonly seen in chronic back-pain problems than in those of an acute, short-term nature. How does depression develop in these cases? Several psychological theories about the development of depression in chronic back pain focus on the issue of control. People with chronic back pain can begin to feel a loss of control over their lives; they feel *totally controlled by the pain*. As this situation progresses, they become more and more hopeless, which leads to a major depression. Once in this state, the person is unable to change the situation even if possible solutions to the situation exist.

The connection between loss of control and depression has been well documented in animal research with dogs. In one experiment two groups of dogs were given electrical shock. One group was warned by a buzzer that the shock was coming while the second group was not warned. The group of dogs who were warned exhibited pretty much their normal behavior. This included whining and howling in response to the shock but otherwise behaving as usual. The other group of dogs (no warning) showed greatly disturbed behavior all of the time, including whining, shaking, and so on, even when the shock was off. This was because they never knew when the shock would come.

In another experiment using electrical shock and dogs, one group was given a series of shocks they could not predict or avoid. Initially the dogs howled and tried to escape each time they were shocked. After a while these dogs laid down and waited for the shocks to occur. At this point, when the shocks would occur, the dogs would simply whine and howl passively, making no attempt to escape (i.e., showing symptoms of depression).

The second part of this experiment is even more telling. The dogs were then placed in an area where they *could* avoid the shock by jumping over a short platform. Normal dogs, who had not been shocked without escape beforehand, quickly learned that they could avoid the shock by escaping. The dogs from the uncontrollable-shock experiment continued to accept the shock in a passive manner, even though an escape route was now available. This occurred even after the experimenter literally dragged the dogs over the platform in an attempt to show them how to escape the shock.

A theory of depression, called the *learned helplessness theory,* was developed based on this animal research. Basically it states that depression is a state of learned helplessness in which the individual "learns" that its behavior has no effect on things that happen around it (or in it, such as pain). Hence these individuals become passive, hopeless, and helpless, much like the dogs in the second experiment. This continues even when the possibility of increased control and "escape" presents itself.

These two experiments and the learned helplessness theory illustrate what we often see in depression and chronic back pain. Patients will often complain that they feel no sense of control or predictability of the pain. In addition, when the pain comes, they feel they are totally at its mercy. A natural consequence of this perceived loss of control is learned helplessness and depression.

Treatment for depression is often appropriate as part of back-pain rehabilitation. Ideally this will include giving the person more of a sense of control over the pain and reassurance about the benign nature of the pain. Psychological pain management can be useful in this regard to help the patient examine the types of thoughts ("catastrophic thoughts") that are part of the depression. Also antidepressant medication can be useful in many cases of major depression. As we have discussed previously, these medicines also appear to have an independent effect on the chronic back pain in terms of pain relief.

Anxiety

In our clinical experience it appears that anxiety about the back pain occurs in the subacute stage. The subacute phase occurs after the acute phase but before the chronic stage. It usually occurs at about the three- to six-month range. At the acute stage the person with back pain generally feels a reasonable sense of hope that the pain will resolve within the near future. As we have seen in previous chapters, in the vast majority of back-pain episodes, this is an accurate belief.

In the subacute phase and at the beginning of the chronic phase, one's thoughts and emotions about the back pain begin to change. It is not uncommon for the person to begin to wonder, "Will this pain ever go away?" "This must be something serious," and "I'll never get better." These types of thoughts lead to anxiety.

Anxiety can occur at different intensities, all the way from nervousness to full panic attacks. Anxiety is generally characterized by the following:

- Muscle tension, including shakiness, jitteriness, trembling, muscle aches, fatigue, restlessness, and inability to relax

- Nervous system overactivity, including sweaty palms, heart racing, dry mouth, upset stomach, diarrhea, lump in throat, shortness of breath, and so on

- Apprehensive expectations, including anxiety, worry, fear, anticipation of misfortune

- Trouble concentrating, including distractability, insomnia, feeling "on edge," irritability, and impatience.

Although most patients believe that their anxiety will subside "when the pain goes away," the anxiety is very often causing a significant increase in pain perception. This results in a vicious cycle of pain, anxiety, more pain, and more anxiety.

As an example of this, Dr. Deardorff recently evaluated and treated a seventy-two-year-old woman who had been scheduled to undergo spine surgery. She was clearly a good candidate for the surgery given all appropriate factors (see chapter 12). As one part of her pain problem, she also had a significant amount of general anxiety. She had been involved in a few sessions of psychological preparation for surgery, which we will often do with anxious or depressed patients. Approximately two weeks prior to the scheduled surgery the patient's leg pain completely disappeared! Her findings on the MRI continued to be abnormal. The surgeon could only explain it under the category of "an act of nature one does not want to argue with." Given this experience, the patient expected that her anxiety and depression would also abate shortly thereafter. To her dismay this did not occur. She continued to be emotional and began to address those issues in psychotherapy.

This is certainly an unusual and rare example, but it does illustrate that removal of the pain does not necessarily mean emotional issues will also then resolve. To wait until the back pain is gone before addressing emotional issues is a trap that will prevent a return to a normal life.

Fear and Phobia

Recent research suggests that fear may be a significant component in back pain. This fear is usually focused on the fear of further injury, increased pain, or both. This fear can be closely linked with anxiety, which is discussed in the previous section.

Fear in back pain is *unreasonable* when it is either not appropriate to the situation or is beyond what it should be given the nature of the situation. This might include being fearful of reinjury when there is no indication that this will occur. When fear is at these levels and interferes with normal functioning, it is considered to be a phobia. A phobia is defined as an irrational fear of an object, activity, or situation causing the person to avoid the object, activity, or situation (e.g., movement).

A new area of scientific investigation in back pain is kinesophobia, or fear of movement. In our clinical practice we see kinesophobia quite routinely. These patients have guarding, slow, and deliberate movements, as well as extreme cautiousness. This is often due not to the pain but rather to a phobia of injury, reinjury, or acute exacerbation.

One case was a forty-two-year-old man who was a very successful lawyer. He had one episode of fairly severe back pain, somewhat localized, which lasted for quite some time. He attributed the onset of the pain to "moving a certain way" while getting out of his car. This had occurred about four months prior to the patient coming to our clinic. In that time he had been seen by several specialists, at least one of whom had recommended spine surgery. The patient came in with extremely slow, almost robotlike movements in an attempt to keep his spine as straight as possible. For fear of making the pain worse, he would not bend. He had developed a very structured ritual in order to get dressed each morning. This included putting his underwear and pants on the floor, stepping into them, and then gradually working them on with the help of a reaching device. He had developed similar rituals for putting his shoes on, driving, working at his desk, and interacting with his children. We ultimately involved him in an aggressive physical-therapy program for reactivation and mobility as well as psychological pain management to address his kinesophobia. We even employed such unusual techniques as having him do a type of obstacle course through the gym with a time clock so that he could not focus on his fear of the pain. There was no medical reason for him to fear the pain or to be a surgical candidate. The patient responded very well to the program with a return to normal activities.

Kinesophobia can cause great problems over the long term. The fear of movement results in the patient attempting to move as little as possible. This guarding behavior causes the muscles in the back to fall into a state of disuse and atrophy. The muscles become weak and tight (shortened) due to lack of use. Any attempt to increase activity will then cause an increase in pain due to the weak and tight muscles. This scares the patient into not doing anything (see figure 14-3). Working through this period of increased pain under supervision with reassurance is critical to recovery from the pain problem.

Anger

Anger is frequently an integral component of chronic back-pain problems. It may be felt and expressed directly or indirectly. We are all familiar with the direct expression of anger. This might include such things as a short temper, irritability, and

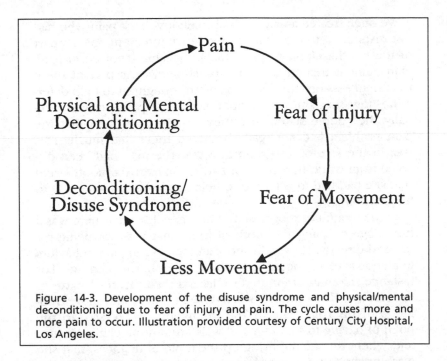

Figure 14-3. Development of the disuse syndrome and physical/mental deconditioning due to fear of injury and pain. The cycle causes more and more pain to occur. Illustration provided courtesy of Century City Hospital, Los Angeles.

explosive behavior, among other things. Indirect anger may be expressed in a number of ways. For instance depression has been defined as "anger turned inward" and may in some cases be a type of indirect anger. We often see back-pain cases where there is no overt anger but an increase in self-destructive behaviors, such as increased smoking, coffee intake, risk taking, and substance abuse (alcohol and/or medicines). These patterns can indicate indirect anger.

Another expression of indirect anger is called passive-aggressiveness. This is anger expressed outwardly but in a passive, indirect manner. An example of this includes an increase in pain (or pain behaviors) in response to someone you are actually angry at. We commonly see this pattern in marital or family relationships. Usually the person with back pain who is expressing anger through increased pain does so unintentionally and is not aware of the pattern.

We once treated a man with chronic low back pain who had not responded to the usual conservative interventions. As part of the multidisciplinary program he became involved in pain-management treatment with a psychologist. As part of these treatment sessions the spouse is often brought in to help determine how the family is responding to the pain problem. Initially the couple stated that they "rarely fight" and that the pain problem had not really bothered them that much. This was in the face of also reporting that the man had been disabled from work, they had not had sex in over six months, and that she had had to get a job to help support the family due to his disability.

As the treatment progressed, it became clear that there was a high degree of anger in both of them that was not being expressed directly. He would show an increase in pain behaviors in response to any possible area of conflict in the marriage. For instance she once attempted to discuss their financial status in the session. He eventually started having more and more trouble with his back pain as the discussion progressed, to the point of having to stand up and walk around the clinic. He also felt, whenever she did bring up the topic of finances, that she was implying that he was bringing all this misery to the family on purpose. In contrast she stated she was simply trying to "brainstorm" about how to realistically manage their finances.

She would also express her anger at the situation indirectly. At first she was very supportive in helping with more responsibilities around the house due to his pain problem. But as the pain went on and on, she became more frustrated with the situation. She started to spend more and more time away from home and away from him. He began to respond to this by unconsciously showing more pain behaviors in order to try to get her attention once again. Of course this drove her farther away. The cycle was becoming worse and worse until the issue was openly discussed in the pain-management sessions.

Entitlement

Another aspect of anger in back pain is that of entitlement. This is a fancy term for the feeling that "somebody or something owes me something for the pain that I am experiencing." We often see this sense of entitlement in cases where the back pain has started as the result of a work-related injury, car accident, or some other injury. People commonly feel they are "entitled" to a pain-free existence and that any limitation of normal activities due to pain is unacceptable. They feel that if their lives are disrupted or limited in any way due to pain, then "somebody should pay." Although in a legal sense this might in part be accurate, from a psychological perspective this attitude can be very self-destructive.

Excessive focus on what you are "entitled to" due to your pain can prevent you from taking responsibility for getting better. When there is litigation involved, the situation becomes even more complex, as we shall see in the next section. Even when there is not litigation involved, human beings will naturally look for a place to "put the blame" for their pain. We do this in an attempt to explain the pain and to express our anger at something. This blaming may be directed at a spouse, doctors who were unable to find a reason for the pain or provide a cure, "the guy who hit me," "the idiot who left a slippery floor for me to fall on," or "God, for putting me in this painful situation." Focusing on *blaming* is a form of entitlement, and it is not healthy for a recovery from back pain.

The most important thing to remember about entitlement is that it is a natural response to extended pain and disability; but if it is not adequately dealt with, it can completely interfere with recovery.

CHANGING YOUR THOUGHTS AND EMOTIONS

Thoughts, Feelings, and Behaviors

A model for understanding how thoughts, emotions, and behaviors interact has been developed by such cognitive researchers as Dr. Aaron Beck, Dr. Albert Ellis, and others. This model (and the method for changing your thoughts) has been termed the ABCDE model and it can be a very useful tool in dealing with back pain. The specifics of the ABCDE model will be discussed shortly, but it is important to have an understanding of how thoughts and emotions operate.

We would all agree that we constantly have thoughts and images going through our head related to evaluating the world around us. In addition we are constantly evaluating the sensations that are going on inside of us as well. These thoughts have been termed automatic thoughts because they often occur automatically, almost out of our awareness. Automatic thoughts have the characteristics of being very fast, virtually out of awareness or unconscious, and highly believable. As we shall see shortly, automatic thoughts have great power over our emotions and behaviors.

Many of the cognitive researchers have also noticed that human beings under stress have a tendency to engage in negative automatic thoughts. Back pain can be a particularly stressful event, easily resulting in a cascade of negative automatic thoughts. Based on these findings, the ABCDE model was developed. The ABCDE stands for the following:

A is the **Activating Event or Antecedent Event,** which is simply the event to which you are responding. This could be an outside event, such as sitting in a traffic jam, or an internal event, such as a severe back spasm.

B is your automatic thought or **Belief** about the activating event. For instance your belief about being in the traffic jam might be "Oh no, this is awful. I will never make the meeting in time. I should have left earlier." Alternatively your belief might be "There's nothing I can do about this traffic jam. I'll take this time to listen to the radio and be as relaxed as possible. I'll leave earlier in the future."

In the back-pain example your automatic thoughts might be "I'll never get better. My back is getting worse and worse. I'll end up a cripple." On the other hand your thoughts about the back pain might be "This pain doesn't mean I'm getting worse. This is usually a temporary thing. I am getting better overall. This pain is nothing to be frightened of."

In each of the above examples the first set of thoughts are *negative automatic thoughts* and the second set of thoughts are *coping* or *rational thoughts*. The difference in the makeup of these thoughts can certainly be seen and will be discussed more fully in a later section.

C is the **Consequent Emotion** that results from the automatic thoughts. Most people think that A causes C, but in reality, C is caused by B. *A person's emotional response to a situation is caused by his or her beliefs about the situation and not by the situation itself.*

D is the **Disputing Thoughts** that are used to change automatic negative thoughts. These are used to help change the way a person thinks about stressful situations (such as back pain) from a negative standpoint to a coping standpoint. In working with patients on doing this exercise, we like to term this process *the power of realistic thinking.*

E is the **Evaluation** part of using the disputing thoughts to challenge the negative automatic thoughts. This process will be discussed further.

The following examples will help you understand just how the ABCDE model operates.

EXAMPLE 1

Activating Event:	You experience a mild increase in your heart rate and feel "uncomfortable and jittery."
Belief:	I'm having a heart attack!!!
Consequent Emotion:	Fear, anxiety, panic.
Resulting Behavior:	Call doctor or go to emergency room.

In this situation the symptoms are being interpreted as a possible heart attack. The subsequent emotions and behavior follow from this belief. Suppose an alternative belief was that

"I just drank four cups of coffee and the caffeine is causing the symptoms." With this explanation the emotions and resulting behavior would be entirely different.

EXAMPLE 2

Activating Event:	You hear a noise at the bedroom window in the middle of the night.
Belief:	There is an intruder trying to get in.
Consequent Emotion:	Fear, panic.
Resulting Behavior:	Call police, hide, grab a weapon.

Again, in this example, the emotions and behavior follow from the belief that there is danger. If alternatively the belief was that the noise was caused by the wind blowing a tree branch against the window, the emotional response and behaviors would be entirely different.

It should be noted that in each of these examples the situations prompting the beliefs are exactly the same. The only difference is how the information is interpreted by the person in terms of beliefs. These beliefs are what caused the emotional response and behavior, not the situation itself!

We often see a similar occurrence in back-pain cases. Take, for instance, the following example:

Activating Event:	Back or neck pain
Beliefs:	"There is something seriously wrong with my spine."
	"My spine is weak and fragile."
	"My pain is going to get worse and worse."
	"I can't cope with this pain."
	"I'll never get better."
	"I'll always have pain."
	"I should be better by now."

	"I should never have let this happen." "My back pain is all their fault." "Nobody really understands my pain." "If I move the wrong way, I'll do myself in."
Consequent Emotion:	Hopelessness Helplessness Anxiety and fear Depression Anger
Resulting Behavior:	Bed rest Social isolation Irritability Physical deconditioning Decreased sex drive Disability from work Use of pain medicines Groaning, moaning, and grimacing Slow, robotic movements

These examples illustrate how our thoughts influence our emotions and behavior. But how can you use this information to help with back pain? This is done through the use of the "three-column" and the "five-column" techniques. The power in using this approach comes from changing your negative automatic thoughts to "realistic, coping, and nurturing" thoughts. By changing your thoughts about the back pain you can change your emotional responses and behaviors.

The Three- and Five-Column Techniques
The ABC and ABCDE can be utilized in a three- and five-column technique. A three-column worksheet can be seen in figure 14-4.

THE THREE-COLUMN TECHNIQUE

Activating Event	Beliefs	Consequent Emotions
Sitting at work. Supervisor gave me too much to do. I'm noticing worse pain in my back as well as in my neck.	"There is something seriously wrong with my back." "My spine is weak and fragile." "If I move the wrong way, I'll do myself in."	Fear
	"I'll never lead a normal life." "I can't cope with this pain."	Helplessness
	"There is nothing I can do about this pain."	Hopelessness
	"My back pain is all their fault." "My boss doesn't understand my pain." "My boss expects too much from me."	Anger and Entitlement
	"I should be better by now." "I should never have let myself get injured in the first place." "This pain is ruining my family."	Guilt

Figure 14.4. Example of the three-column technique.

The three columns represent the A, B, and C event discussed above. It is useful to make several copies of the ABC worksheet in order to practice identifying activating events, beliefs, and consequent emotions. The three-column technique is a tool to enable you essentially to run the automatic negative thoughts in slow motion. You can use the three-column technique to analyze your thoughts and feelings whenever a stressful situation presents itself.

An activating event can be any stressor, such as back pain, a situation, a memory, or an interaction with another person. At first it can be difficult to "flesh out" the beliefs or automatic negative thoughts about a situation. Automatic negative thoughts often contain such words as *should, ought, must, never,* and *always.* As can be seen in the above example, phrases with these words are common in negative thinking.

Negative thinking also takes on certain styles, as discussed by Ellen Mohr Catalano in her book entitled *The Chronic Pain Control Workbook.* Briefly these styles can be summarized as follows:

Catastrophizing
This type of negative thinking is characterized by imagining the worst possible scenario and then acting as if that will actually happen. It will often include a series of *What if*s such as:

"What if I never get better?"

"What if I get worse?"

"What if I become a cripple?"

"What if . . . ?"

In catastrophic thinking, the dire predictions are not based on facts but rather on pessimistic beliefs.

Magnifying or Filtering
This negative-thinking style involves focusing on only the negative aspects of a situation to the exclusion of any positive elements or options. This style will commonly include searching for evidence of "how bad things really are" and discounting any positive or coping focus. Examples include:

"There is nothing that will help my back pain."

"Everything in my life is rotten due to this pain."

"Nobody really cares."

"The doctors have nothing to offer."

"I've tried everything, and nothing has helped at all."

This style of negative thinking is often characterized by discounting and "yes-butting." No matter what positive option or coping method is suggested, the back-pain sufferer will discount it with a "yes-but." For instance a person with back pain has been able to stop the pain medicines and start on a mild exercise program. When this is discussed as being a very positive change, the person retorts "Yes, but I still have pain, I haven't returned to work, and I'll bet this pain doesn't go away." This type of thinking continues to foster helplessness, hopelessness, and depression.

Black-and-White Thinking
This type of thinking is seeing things either one way or the other. There is no middle ground or shades of gray. This type of thinking is typified by

"Either I'm cured or I'm not."

"I either have pain or I don't."

"The treatment either works or it doesn't."

"This doctor is either good or bad."

This type of thinking undermines any small steps toward improvement, severely limits one's options, and filters out any positive aspects of the back-pain situation.

Overgeneralizing
This is the process of taking one aspect of a situation and applying it to all other situations. It involves generalizing reac-

tions to situations in which such reactions are not appropriate. For instance:

"With this back pain there's no way I could handle going to a movie."

"People don't want to be around me with this back pain."

"My wife told me to try to do something about the pain. She must be ready to leave the marriage."

As can be seen, this style of irrational thinking will take one incident and make it apply to many other situations.

Mind Reading
This negative-thinking trap involves making assumptions about what other people are thinking without actually knowing. The person will then act on these assumptions, which are usually erroneous. Examples of this might include the following:

"I know my wife thinks I'm less of a man due to this pain."

"I know my husband thinks I'm exaggerating."

"My doctor doesn't really think I'll get better even though she tells me I will."

"They're not telling me everything about my pain problem."

If you accept these assumptions as facts, then your behavior will follow accordingly, and you will create a possible self-fulfilling prophecy. For example, your spouse might ask, "How does your back feel today?" Instead of taking his or her comment at face value, you believe he or she really means "Are you still letting that little back pain bother you?" So you respond, "How do think it feels today! The same as always, that's how." You can easily guess how this scenario would be completed.

*Should*s

Should statements are key elements in negative automatic thinking. Examples of such thinking include

"I should be getting better."

"I should never have allowed this to happen."

"I should have known not to have that spine surgery."

"My employer should have protected my back better."

"I should be tougher."

"My family should be more helpful."

Should thinking also includes terms such as *ought, must, always,* and *never. Should* thinking is very judgmental and often involves measuring your performance against some irrational perfect standard. It has the effect of making you feel worthless, useless, and inadequate. When directed at others, it will have the effect of making you feel angry and resentful in those relationships.

Blaming

In blaming, the person makes something or someone else responsible for the back pain. This type of negative thinking is very often seen in cases of industrial injury, automobile accidents, or other such trauma. Examples include

"My boss is to blame for my pain. If . . ."

"They should have swept up that water I slipped on. It's all their fault."

"That guy who hit me owes me everything for the pain I'm suffering."

"I'm to blame for this lousy back-pain problem."

Blaming as a form of irrational thinking can be focused either externally or internally. Blaming can be very destructive in keeping you from focusing on what you need to do to get better.

ATTACKING AND CHANGING NEGATIVE AUTOMATIC THOUGHTS

Once you have identified an activating event, you can then identify either the beliefs about the situation or the emotions you are experiencing. Often it is easier to identify your emotional reactions first and then work backward to identify the negative automatic thoughts or beliefs.

When you have become good at identifying the ABC components of stress and pain, you will expand the three-column technique to a five-column technique. This is done by adding the columns for Disputing Thoughts and Evaluation. The disputing thoughts are constructed to directly "attack" and counter the negative automatic thoughts that are generated in column B. The Evaluation column is then used to record how these disputing thoughts have affected the original negative thoughts, the emotions, and the overall stress of the situation. Figure 14.5 is an extension of the preceding three-column example and illustrates the entire process.

As you practice with this technique, you will find it to be a very powerful tool in decreasing your negative emotional responses to stressful situations including pain. Further resources for this technique are given in the bibliography.

OTHER FACTORS THAT INFLUENCE PAIN, SUFFERING, AND DISABILITY

Positive Reinforcement of Pain Behavior
Pain behaviors are the behaviors that help us communicate to others around us that we are experiencing pain. These might include such things as talking about the pain, taking pain medicine, yelling out, grimacing, groaning, moving slowly, and being very silent. It is only by these types of behaviors that others

can try to gauge our level of pain experience. Pain is an individual experience that cannot be directly measured, so we use pain behaviors to communicate our distress.

Any behavior that we exhibit can be reinforced by those around us. Further, any behavior that is reinforced will increase in frequency (by definition). For example simple research studies have shown that if you get a classroom of students to pay attention to the teacher each time she moves to the left side of the classroom and ignore her when she is on the right side, after a while she will be teaching the entire class from the left side of the room. Even more interesting is that the teacher will not be aware that this reinforcement of being on the left side of the classroom is even occurring! The reader can probably think of a variety of behaviors that are reinforced throughout the day, including working for a paycheck, recreational activities, family interactions, and so on.

As with any behavior, pain behavior can also be reinforced by the environment around us, and this most commonly occurs in the family setting. This reinforcement can be very direct and obvious, such as asking to rub your spouse's back when a groan is heard, "knowing" when to bring pain medication even when your spouse has not asked simply by "the look on his face," or warning him not to "overdo it" when you see him slowly limping past you. These are examples of direct attention (reinforcement) for pain behaviors. This reinforcement can also be quite subtle, as can be seen in the following example given by Dr. Fordyce, the pioneer in this area of pain research: "The pain-ridden wife walks across the room without displaying pain and her paper-reading husband does not look up. When she limps, holds her back, or gasps while walking, his attention is diverted to her, and he watches and perhaps makes a solicitous comment."

Dr. Fordyce also gives an extreme but not uncommon example of how powerful direct reinforcement can be. The patient was a man in his forties who had been incapacitated for nearly twenty years. His wife worked to supplement his disability income. The husband was completely deactivated, spending most of his time in bed watching TV. She would prepare din-

THE FIVE-COLUMN TECHNIQUE

Activating Event	Beliefs	Consequent Emotions	Disputing Thoughts	Evaluation
Sitting at work. Supervisor gave me too much to do. I'm noticing worse pain in my back as well as in my neck.	"There is something seriously wrong with my back." "My spine is weak and fragile." "If I move the wrong way, I'll do myself in."	Fear	"Hurt does not equal harm! This pain does not mean injury." "The spine is a strong structure." "I am not at risk for injury."	Much less fear
	"I'll never lead a normal life." "I can't cope with this pain."	Helplessness	No one can predict the future." "I'm learning ways to cope. I've made it through before."	More feeling of control
	"There is nothing I can do about this pain."	Hopelessness	"There are things I can do. They are . . ."	Somewhat better
	"My back pain is all their fault." "My boss doesn't understand my pain." "My boss expects too much from me."	Anger and Entitlement	"Blaming does not help me get better." "My boss acts that way toward everyone." "I can get a lot done if I work steadily and pace myself."	Mild decrease in anger
	"I should be better by now." "I should never have let myself get injured in the first place." "This pain is ruining my family."	Guilt	"I am trying to get better and am working hard at it." "It was not my fault." "There are things I can do to lead a quality life regardless of the pain."	Guilt improved

Figure 14.5. Expansion of the three-column technique to five columns.

ner for him in the evenings and bring it to the bedroom. When he would make an attempt to get out of bed to eat in another room or socialize with friends, his wife would chastise him for taking such risks. Her nurturing behavior was actually being reinforced by his decrease in pain behaviors each time she attended to him. In addition, his pain behaviors were continually reinforced by her attention to them. It is similar to parents who indulge a whining child. The indulgent behavior is reinforced by the temporary cessation of the child's whining while the whining is reinforced over the long term by continued attention from the parents.

Direct reinforcement of pain behaviors can increase both disability and suffering, which in turn increases one's perception of pain. It is important to note that direct reinforcement of pain behaviors (as with the other influences to be discussed subsequently) are most likely to have influences in the chronic-pain stages, after most tissue healing has occurred. This is usually considered to be important four to six months after the onset of pain.

Avoidance Learning
Behavior can also be influenced by what has been termed avoidance learning. This is behavior that we engage in to "avoid" consequences that are negative or aversive. In this way those behaviors are actually being reinforced. Avoidance learning can also influence pain behaviors. In this scenario certain behaviors will be reinforced in an attempt to avoid the pain. Dr. Fordyce gives the following examples:

A certain limp or posture is found to be effective in being more comfortable and to avoid the pain. Thus it is reinforced each time it is rehearsed and becomes part of the person's usual behavior.

Bed rest is found to decrease the pain. Thus in order to avoid any pain, the person spends more and more time in bed. Anytime an increase in activity is attempted, the pain increases more and more due to weakening of muscles and other factors. Attempts at becoming more active are punished by increased pain, and bed rest is reinforced by avoidance learning.

A patient may know that walking more than three hundred yards has resulted in increased pain in the past. Therefore whenever this goal is approached, the expectation for increased pain occurs. The patient will then avoid coming near the three-hundred-yard mark in the walking program.

Early in the history of a pain problem a limp is reinforced by avoiding pain, as in the above example. After some time the limp itself leads to reinforcing from family members and others (e.g., "Let me help you," "I'll take care of that," and "Don't walk all that way, I'll drive you," etc.). At this point in time, it may not be necessary for pain to occur for the person to limp. It is an independent behavior in and of itself.

These examples illustrate in simple terms what is actually a complex and subtle process. Another area that has received great attention in research recently is avoidance learning as it relates to job dissatisfaction and lack of recovery from back pain. In the Boeing Study, researchers at the University of Washington found that one of the strongest predictors of whether a worker would have prolonged back-injury disability was job dissatisfaction. One would think it might be something like heavy work, bending, problems with one's spine, or some other "physical" explanation. This was not the case.

It is important to underscore the fact that the person who is experiencing the pain, as well as his or her family members, is usually completely unaware of these influences of reinforcement and avoidance learning.

Reinforcement by the Medical Community
Dr. Fordyce also points out that the medical community can actually foster pain behavior and disability in the following ways:

- Attention from physicians or other health care providers
- The use of pain medications
- The restriction of exercise and activity

The first of these factors is fairly straightforward. It simply includes the attention that one receives from the medical community when seeking treatment for a chronic pain problem. We have treated many chronic-pain patients who clearly obtain a type of nurturance from their relationships with various aspects of the medical community. This might include such things as seeing the physical therapist a few times per week for hot packs and massage, visiting the doctor on a frequent basis, or going into the hospital occasionally for management of a pain "flare-up." We will often see this pattern of reinforcement in patients who have very few other areas of reinforcement. An example of this might be the person who has lost his job due to pain and has few supportive family relationships and no recreational interests. In this scenario (which we see commonly) the pain problem and its treatment is virtually the center of the person's life.

The use of pain medications can be a powerful reinforcer for pain behavior. This topic is fully explored in chapter 11 and will only be briefly mentioned here. Pain medications are often prescribed on a "prn" (as-needed). Under this prescription, pain medications are given when the person is experiencing pain (showing pain behaviors) and are not given when there are no pain behaviors. This method would appear to make common sense, but it can actually set up strong influences over pain behavior. Pain medication is in no way a treatment for a back problem; rather it is used while a solution is being sought. Pain medication provides pain relief as well as an improved sense of emotional well-being. This improved sense of well-being might include such things as relief from anxiety, a general sense of relaxation, or improved energy and sleep in the person who is depressed.

Given the fact that pain medicine is very reinforcing, pain behaviors can quickly come under their influence. This occurs because the person must usually demonstrate pain behaviors in order to justify the request for pain medicines. The pain medicines are then taken, which in turn reinforce the pain behaviors. As the pain becomes more chronic, the likelihood of pain behaviors being reinforced by pain-medicine use becomes greater and greater. Physicians will often play a role in this process as apparent solutions to the pain problem become fewer and fewer. A common response is to "Do something!", which unfortunately often means throwing more pain medications at the problem. The correct method of prescribing pain medication for back-pain problems is discussed in chapter 11.

The medical community can also inadvertently reinforce back-pain behaviors in how it manages bed rest and activity. As discussed throughout this book, the prescription for extended bed rest for back pain is common. This is often followed by the admonition to "let the pain be your guide" in terms of activity. In the majority of cases, as the back pain becomes more chronic, this type of approach will actually make the entire problem worse, not better. This simply reinforces the entire sick role in both the patient and those around him or her. It also creates much of the unnecessary disability we see with chronic back-pain sufferers.

Difficulty Coping with Being Well

As Dr. M. Scott Peck has stated so eloquently and succinctly in his book *The Road Less Traveled,* "Life is difficult." In some cases of longer-term back pain, our multidisciplinary assessment will reveal that part of the pain problem relates to the patient not being able to cope with being well. The reader's first response to such a notion may be "That's crazy!!!! Who would not want to be well?" This is not a conscious decision on the part of the patient. Rather the stress of coping with being well is more negative than focusing on the back pain and living in the sick role. Thus the back pain actually shelters the patient from stress, responsibility demands, and other aspects of normal everyday life. In these cases it is important to assess the "cost" (in psychological, physical, and emotional terms) for the person to actually get better. The following example will help illustrate this point:

Mr. T. was a fifty-three-year-old railroad conductor who injured his back while attempting to throw a large railroad track switch. He had been through the usual course of physical therapy, but his back pain continued. He had an MRI that revealed a slight disc bulge, but the doctors did not think these findings accounted for his level of pain. He had been disabled from work for approximately twelve months at the time of our assessment. As with the previous doctors the physical evaluation revealed little that would account for his pain. However, the psychological evaluation revealed several things that helped explain his pain. First, he had been experiencing more and more stress in the work setting just prior to the injury. He had a new boss who was constantly "on" him. The patient was very concerned about his ability to do the job given his age and the number of younger people who were ready to take his place. He feared his new boss was trying to "get rid of" him. In addition the railroad disability program allowed him to collect 80 percent of his full pay while he was disabled. He might also be eligible for early medical retirement or retraining if the back pain did not resolve.

This example clearly indicates that the "cost" for this patient to get better was to return to a job that was becoming more and more stressful, return to a job he might be fired from, lose the possibility of retraining, and give up 80 percent of his pay for being in a less stressful (albeit painful) situation. It should be clearly understood that this situation does not show malingering or faking. It is just a situation of many pressures operating on this person's back-pain problem. The pain situation protected him from another situation that for him was even worse.

Another less extreme example is as follows: Sharon is a thirty-year-old woman who has been rather "sickly" since childhood. She had back pain that seemed to "come out of nowhere" and had been with her for the past two years. She had been through a variety of evaluation and treatment approaches, which were of little help. She would consistently report some relief at the beginning of treatment, but the pain would eventually return to its usual levels. Our evaluation revealed that Sharon had a very inconsistent work history, a history of a number of failed relationships, and little in the way of social involvement. The last two years had been almost entirely focused on her back-pain problem in terms of going to doctors, therapists, and other healers. It was clear that the back pain was helping to distract her from other very stressful aspects of her life and sheltering her from the demands of normal functioning. The cost for her to become well would have been very great without help in other areas of her life. Although she was very depressed and anxious in her chronic back-pain problem, the other prospects were certainly no better. Until she was able to focus on these issues, her back pain would not resolve.

Conclusions

In thinking about your own back-pain problem, it is important to assess whether the pain is being influenced by any of the factors discussed above. To summarize, these include factors in many areas of the pain system including nociception, thoughts, emotions, pain sensation, suffering, pain behaviors, and the psychosocial environment. It is important to acknowledge the power that emotions can have on one's back pain including

- Depression

- Anxiety

- Fear and phobia

- Anger

- Entitlement

The longer the pain lingers, the more likely one or more of these emotions is increasing the pain. Using the ABCDE method can help manage the negative thoughts and emotions that often occur with back pain.

Lastly, the influence of nonphysical factors on back pain, disability, and suffering must be acknowledged. There are very few doctors who will take these factors into account, even though recent research indicates they may be among the most important in chronic back-pain cases. These factors include

- Positive reinforcement from others of the pain
- Avoidance learning to "avoid" the possibility of pain
- Reinforcement of pain and suffering by the medical community
- Having difficulty coping with being well

If any of these influences are part of the pain problem, the back pain will not resolve until it is addressed. Being aware and accepting that these factors are occurring is the first step in becoming healthy and deciding to stop suffering because of the pain.

CHAPTER 15

EMOTIONS, BACK PAIN, AND DISABILITY: A SELF-ASSESSMENT APPROACH

In the previous chapter we discovered how many factors can influence your perception of back pain. These include such things as tissue damage or injury, your thoughts about the pain, your emotions, and the environment. This approach to back pain is radically different from that of traditional medicine, which tends to look strictly for something to "fix." As we have discussed many times throughout the book, this traditional approach will often lead to failed treatments, even making the patient worse off than before any treatment at all.

This chapter will focus further on the nontissue, emotional, and environmental aspects of back pain. Hopefully the previous chapters have firmly convinced you that these factors are every bit as important as (or, in our opinion, actually more important than) the "physical" part of back pain. This chapter is organized so that you can self-assess the "nonphysical" aspects of back pain. These factors include general stress, work stress, depression, anxiety, and anger. In addition to assessing these influences it is imperative to search for patterns to your pain and emotions. This is done by using the pain-activity-mood-medication (PAMM) diary. This method will be presented first. Finally, there will be an assessment of your overall disability as a result of your back pain. This will help you determine very specifically how much your back pain is affecting your life and will allow you to assess positive progress as you utilize the approaches we have outlined in this book.

HOW TO USE THIS CHAPTER

We will provide one caveat before you embark on this self-assessment chapter: People with back pain don't like to address these issues. We will universally investigate these issues with patients as part of the multidisciplinary approach. It is very common for patients to say, "I don't want to fill out these questionnaires about my emotions or my back pain." They say that simply filling out the assessments makes them feel worse because it causes them to focus on the pain, suffering, and disability. It is essential to assess and address these issues even though it might be difficult at first. This information will help you determine the intensity of each aspect of your back-pain problem. You can then begin to make changes for the better using the guidelines in this book. Also the assessments can be taken again and again so that you will know how you are improving with your back-pain problem.

As you investigate these other influences on your back pain, it will be important not to think, "If only the back pain were gone, all of these things would be fine." This is a common thought among back-pain sufferers and it is a trap. This type of thinking will prevent taking action to correct the other aspects of your pain problem, which you will self-assess in this chapter and which were discussed in the previous chapter. Very often the cure of a back-pain problem lies in decreasing the focus on pain relief and increasing the focus on the other aspects of suffering.

Time	Activity	Pain Level	Medication	Mood
7:00 A.M.	Awake	5	2 codeine	Anger-5
8:00	Out of bed	6		
9:00	TV	5		Dep.-6
10:00	Walk	8	2 codeine	Frust.-6
11:00	TV	5		
12:00	Lunch	5	2 codeine	
1:00 P.M.		5		

(continued on next page)

282

Time	Activity	Pain Level	Medication	Mood
2:00	Fight with			
3:00	spouse	9	3 codeine	Anger-9
4:00	Cocktails	6	Alcohol	
5:00		6		Dep.-3
6:00		7		
7:00	Dinner	8	2 codeine	
8:00				
9:00	Attempt sex,	5	Sleep meds	
10:00	no good	6	2 codeine	Frust.-9
11:00	TV	7		
12:00	Can't sleep	8	2 codeine	Anger-8
1:00 A.M.	TV	5		
2:00				
3:00	Awake		2 codeine	Anger-9
4:00				
5:00	Awake	8	1 codeine	
6:00				

Figure 15.1. Example of a completed PAMM assessment.

The results of the assessments in this chapter can be used in a variety of ways depending upon your situation. If your back pain has just occurred recently (acute), certain results of the self-assessments can tell you whether you are at risk for developing a chronic back-pain syndrome. If you suffer from chronic back pain, the results can tell you if the emotional aspects of your pain need to be addressed. In addition the results can help you make a better decision if surgery has been recommended. Exactly how to use the results of the self-assessments will be discussed further at the end of the chapter.

THE PAMM AND MIND-BODY AWARENESS

PAMM is our acronym for the pain-activity-mood-medication diary. These are very important elements of your back-pain problem that need to be investigated. Completing a PAMM diary assessment will help you identify patterns in your pain that can aid in diagnosis and treatment, understand the mind-body connection in back pain, and identify improvement in your back-pain problem. Overall, the PAMM assessment information will make you very aware of all aspects of your back-pain problem that might need to be addressed. A sample PAMM assessment can be seen in figure 15-1. The ratings are done as follows: Pain is rated on a scale of 0 (no pain at all) to 10 (worst pain imaginable); Mood is rated on a scale of 0 (no negative emotion) to 10 (very severe emotional upset, such as depression or anger). Activities are abbreviated to allow the person simply to remember the incident. This makes the charting quick, easy, and usable. Medications are listed as they are used (alcohol amounts can be included in this category).

The PAMM assessment can be expanded for the individual's needs, both initially and as improvement occurs. For example you can add cigarette and coffee use, or a column for irrational and rational thoughts, as was done in the previous chapter on suffering. In addition the activity and moods column can be used for both negative and positive activities. This might include accomplishments related to overcoming your pain problem, such as tracking your exercise schedule, charting your positive emotions, writing down your coping thoughts, and monitoring your tapering off of pain medicines.

As can be seen in the PAMM example, this person has several aspects to his or her back-pain problem and has a fully developed chronic pain syndrome. These symptoms include a high level of pain ratings, very little physical activity, very little socializing, stressful interactions with a spouse, problems with sex due to pain, significant pain medication use, often linked with emotional upset, sleep disruption, and general emotional upset throughout the day. This person is experiencing mostly depression ("Dep."), anger, and frustration as part of the back-pain problem.

Research has shown that people have difficulty accurately remembering levels of pain and moods that have occurred as recently as within the last week. The PAMM diary can help track this in a very reliable manner because you record the levels as they occur. You may be able to identify such patterns as follows (possible interpretations are given in parentheses):

- The pain increases over the course of the day, being worse in the evening (a possible muscle tension component).

- The pain is worse at work than at home (possible dissatisfaction and stress at work).

- The pain is better or worse when you are around certain people or certain situations (an emotional aspect to your pain including resentment or anger).

- The pain is better when you are sitting or bending over and worse when you are standing upright and walking (possible spinal stenosis).

- Taking pain medicine or using alcohol when you are not in that much pain but rather when you are emotionally upset (using the medication to calm your emotions).

- Your activities are mostly sitting around the house all day watching TV because you are in "too much pain" (deconditioning syndrome).

- You are feeling better and want to try additional activities, such as a walk around the block or taking a swim. You decide not to because someone involved in your injury lawsuit might see you (the pain and disability are being worsened by the lawsuit).

- The pain and your "pain behaviors" are worse when you are mad at your spouse (using pain to communicate anger or "punish" others indirectly).

The above are only examples, and the possible findings on the PAMM assessment are endless. Once you have used the PAMM diary technique for one or two weeks, you can begin to see exactly where your back-pain problem needs to be attacked. We should state that compliance in doing the PAMM diary can be difficult. You will get out of the diary what you put into it!

WHAT IS STRESS?

Stress has become a very common word in today's vocabulary. Even so it means so many different things to so many different people that its precise definition is unknown to most. To discover what stress means to you, complete the following exercise: "Stress is _____." List at least ten things, situations, or people that result in stress:

Now go back and review your list. Where does your stress come from? Is your stress related to short-term things (e.g., being in a traffic jam) or to long-term things (e.g., your career)? Is most of your stress somehow related to your back pain? In reviewing your list, do most of the stressors appear out of your control?

For the purposes of this discussion, we will define stress as follows: Stress results from dealing with something that places "special" demands on a person. A "special" demand is anything that is considered or perceived to be unusual or out of the ordinary related to the person's usual set of experiences. Stress results from a person's perception of physical or psychological threat.

It is important to notice that stress is an individual experience. Something may be very stressful for one person and an absolute delight to another person. As a simple example, one person may think of going to the beach as a wonderful, relaxing experience that includes lying on the sand, listening to the seagulls, and breathing the ocean air. Another person may consider it an absolute nightmare that conjures up images of sunburn, crowded parking lots, gritty sandwiches full of sand, ants and bugs, seagull droppings, and dirty ocean water. As we saw in the previous chapter, it is not a particular situation that is stressful, it is one's assessment of that situation. Thus your "stress list" will always be unique to you.

Even with these individual differences there do appear to be major stressors that can impact us all. Often we are unaware of the influence of these stressors on our physical well-being (including our back pain) and our emotional state. Major life stressors have been researched extensively by Thomas Holmes, M.D., at the University of Washington School of Medicine beginning in 1967. As a result of this research the Schedule of Recent Experience (SRE) was developed. This assessment consists of life events that constitute stressful changes. Scores on the SRE have been found to relate to a number of health problems, including sudden cardiac death, heart attack, chronic illness, and a host of less serious health problems (e.g., getting a cold or flu). These studies lend support to the idea that life stress increases overall susceptibility to illness including back pain.

SCHEDULE OF RECENT EXPERIENCE

Part A

Instructions. Think back on each possible life event listed below and decide if it happened to you within the last year. If the event did happen, check the box next to it.

	Check here if event happened to you	Mean Value (use for scoring later)
1. A lot more or a lot less trouble with the boss	_____	_____
2. A major change in sleeping habits (sleeping a lot more or a lot less, or change in part of day when asleep)	_____	_____
3. A major change in eating habits (a lot more or a lot less food intake, or very different meal hours or surroundings)	_____	_____
4. A revision of personal habits (dress, manners, association, etc.)	_____	_____
5. A major change in your usual type and/or amount of recreation	_____	_____
6. A major change in your social activities (clubs, dancing, movies, visiting, etc.)	_____	_____
7. A major change in church activities (a lot more or a lot less than usual)	_____	_____
8. A major change in number of family get-togethers (a lot more or a lot less than usual)	_____	_____
9. A major change in financial state (a lot worse off or a lot better off than usual)	_____	_____
10. In-law troubles	_____	_____
11. A major change in the number of arguments with spouse (a lot more or a lot less than usual regarding child rearing, personal habits, etc.)	_____	_____
12. Sexual difficulties	_____	_____

(continued on next page)

288

Part B

Instructions. In the space provided indicate the *number of times* that each applicable event happened to you within the last two years.

	Number of Times ×	Mean Value =	Your Score
13. Major personal injury or illness	_____	_____	_____
14. Death of a close family member (other than spouse)	_____	_____	_____
15. Death of spouse	_____	_____	_____
16. Death of a close friend	_____	_____	_____
17. Gaining a new family member (through birth, adoption, elder moving in, etc.)	_____	_____	_____
18. Major change in the health or behavior of a family member	_____	_____	_____
19. Change in residence	_____	_____	_____
20. Detention in jail or other institution	_____	_____	_____
21. Minor violations of the law (traffic tickets, jaywalking, disturbing the peace, etc.)	_____	_____	_____
22. Major business readjustment (merger, reorganization, bankruptcy, etc.)	_____	_____	_____
23. Marriage	_____	_____	_____
24. Divorce	_____	_____	_____
25. Marital separation from spouse	_____	_____	_____
26. Outstanding personal achievement	_____	_____	_____
27. Son or daughter leaving home (marriage, attending college, etc.)	_____	_____	_____
28. Retirement from work	_____	_____	_____
29. Major change in working hours or conditions	_____	_____	_____
30. Major change in responsibilities at work (promotion, demotion, lateral transfer)	_____	_____	_____
31. Being fired from work	_____	_____	_____

(continued on next page)

	Number of Times ×	Mean Value =	Your Score
32. Major change in living conditions (building a new home, remodeling, deterioration of home or neighborhood)	_____	_____	_____
33. Spouse beginning or ceasing work outside the home	_____	_____	_____
34. Taking on a mortgage greater than $10,000 (purchasing a home, business, etc.)	_____	_____	_____
35. Taking on a mortgage or loan for less than $10,000 (purchasing a car, TV, freezer, etc.)	_____	_____	_____
36. Foreclosure on a mortgage or loan	_____	_____	_____
37. Vacation	_____	_____	_____
38. Changing to a new school	_____	_____	_____
39. Changing to a different line of work	_____	_____	_____
40. Beginning or ceasing formal schooling	_____	_____	_____
41. Marital reconciliation with mate	_____	_____	_____
42. Pregnancy	_____	_____	_____

Total score Part A _____
Total score Part B _____
Overall Total _____

Scoring the SRE

The "mean values" for each life event are listed below. Write in the mean values of those events that happened to you in parts A and B. For the items in part B multiply the mean value by the number of times an event happened and enter the result under "Your score."

Add up the mean values in part A and your scores in part B to get your total score.

Life Event	Mean Value
1	23
2	16
3	15
4	24

5 19
6 18
7 19
8 15
9 38
10 29
11 35
12 39
13 53
14 63
15 100
16 37
17 39
18 44
19 20
20 63
21 11
22 39
23 50
24 73
25 65
26 28
27 29
28 45
29 20
30 29
31 47
32 25
33 26
34 31
35 17
36 30
37 13
38 20
39 36
40 26
41 45
42 40

The more "stress" or change that you have experienced recently, the more likely you are to get sick. Your life-stress score can be analyzed as follows:

0 to 75	Minimal levels
76 to 150	Moderate levels
151 to 299	High levels
300 and above	Severe levels

Source: The Schedule of Recent Experience © 1976. Used by permission of Thomas H. Holmes, M.D., Department of Psychiatry and Behavioral Sciences, University of Washington School of Medicine, Seattle, WA.

As discussed by Drs. Matthew McKay and Martha Davis, of those people with a score over 300 for the past year, almost 80 percent get sick in the near future. Of those with a score 150 to 299, about 50 percent get sick in the near future. Of those with a score of 150 and below, only about 30 percent get sick in the near future. In addition stress can be cumulative. Stressful events from two or more years ago could still be affecting you now. *As you complete the life-stress assessment, you may find that the onset or increase of your back pain correlates with a number of significant life changes.* It should be noted that Dr. Holmes discovered that positive life changes can also be stressful. You may have noticed that such things as marriage, a birth, and an outstanding personal achievement are all "stressful." We will discuss further how this information can also help you recover from your back-pain problem.

WORK STRESS

Another important category of general life stress is work stress. Stress at work appears to be one of the primary influences related to onset of back pain. As was discussed previously, in the Boeing Study one of the most powerful predictors of back disability was job dissatisfaction. It was found that those employees who were generally dissatisfied with their work situation were more likely to remain disabled from a back injury.

Most people spend a good part of their waking hours in some type of work setting. Unfortunately many people are unhappy in their work situation, and this is most often due to some type of relationship(s) with others at work. Dr. Leonard

Felder has written extensively on the issue of work stress. In his most recent book, *Does Someone at Work Treat You Badly?*, he explores the impact of these stressful relationships on a person's mental, emotional, and physical well-being. He developed the following test to help determine if work stress is (or has been) a problem. You need only answer the following questions as honestly as possible. If you are not currently working because of your back pain, answer each question *as it would have applied* during the work you were doing when the back pain caused your disability.

WORK-STRESS ASSESSMENT

1. In the past few weeks or months, have you had difficulties with anyone at work—a boss, coworker, colleague, employee, customer, supplier, or business partner? **Yes No**

2. Do you sometimes dread having to see this person at work or in social situations, or have you ever felt anxious when he or she has called and left a message for you to return the call? **Yes No**

3. Have you begun conversations in your head with this person, or arguments in your mind where you defend yourself or try to explain your side of the conflict? **Yes No**

4. Have you ever been inundated with thoughts about this difficult individual when you are trying to fall asleep, or when you wake up in the middle of the night, or when you are trying to relax on a weekend or a vacation? **Yes No**

5. Do you find yourself second-guessing your own performance or feeling self-critical as a result of your interactions with this unpleasant individual? **Yes No**

6. Is your creativity blocked or your clarity of mind hampered somewhat by the lingering discomfort of having to deal with such a difficult person? **Yes No**

(continued on next page)

WORK-STRESS ASSESSMENT *(continued)*

7. Have you noticed that you have been trying to calm yourself down after work lately by eating more, drinking more, or smoking more than is healthy for you? **Yes No**

8. Are you becoming more impatient or short-tempered at work due to your tensions with this person? **Yes No**

9. Have you become more susceptible lately to colds, flus, stomach problems, or muscle aches in your neck, shoulders, or back? Is it possible that you are carrying a lot of physical tension in your body as a result of the emotional tension you are feeling toward this individual? **Yes No**

10. Do you sometimes feel resentful that this individual treats other people at work a lot better than she or he treats you? **Yes No**

11. Do you find yourself wondering why you are sometimes singled out for criticism or harsh treatment while at the same time you haven't been acknowledged by this individual for the things you've done well? **Yes No**

12. Have you begun to dislike your job or have you thought about quitting as a result of this unpleasant situation with a difficult individual? **Yes No**

13. Have you noticed that you are more irritable or impatient with your spouse or lover, or with your children or your friends as a result of your leftover frustrations from your situations at work? **Yes No**

14. Is your paycheck or your financial security being jeopardized by the unresolved tensions between you and this person? **Yes No**

15. Have you let some projects go sour or lost some good opportunities for advancement because you are unable to overcome the obstacles put up by this unpleasant individual? **Yes No**

16. Are you feeling discouraged that this person has continued to treat you badly despite your efforts to improve the situation? **Yes No**

Scoring of the Work-Stress Assessment

Scoring is done by adding up the number of times you answered yes to the questions. Remember, if you are not currently working, complete the questions for your previous job or the job you were doing when the back pain occurred. After you have totaled the "Yes" responses, see which of the following groups you fall into:

Number of Items	Work-Stress Category
0	No work stress
1–5	Moderate—This constitutes either the beginning of a work-stress situation or an ongoing mild level of work stress.
6–10	Severe—This is a serious level of work stress and is (or was) causing you significant emotional and physical distress.

Source: Self-Test of Work Stress © 1993. Used by permission of Leonard Felder, Ph.D., from *Does Someone at Work Treat You Badly?*, Berkley Publishing Group.

In our clinical work with back-pain patients, work stress often appears to have influenced the onset of the pain problem *and* the person's ability to get well. In some situations the work setting is so stressful that we advise the patient that it is unlikely that his or her back pain will resolve until the situation is changed or the person's coping skills are increased dramatically. In these cases the back pain is one way the body is telling the person that the work stress is virtually intolerable.

It is our belief that unless these issues are addressed, there is a decreased chance of the back pain resolving regardless of the treatment. You can think of this in terms of "the cost of getting better." If your "reward" for improving your functioning, not living like a back-pain victim, and getting beyond your back-pain problem is to return to a job that you can't stand, it is highly unlikely your pain will go away. This is why such groups as jet-fighter pilots and professional athletes involved in serious accidents causing back injuries are very rarely disabled from their occupations. Their drive and motivation to return to work, in addition to the satisfaction they get from their work, is incredibly high. This allows the body to heal faster, prevents chronic pain from developing, and helps the mind "turn off" the pain. If the thought of returning to work is less than appealing to you, your mind may be using the pain to prevent you from having to deal with this stress.

If you scored highly on the above assessment, work stress may have played (or is playing) a key role in the pain. Unless the situation is changed, continuing the search for treatments for your back pain will probably be in vain.

DEPRESSION

As discussed in the previous chapter, depression is a very common experience in more long-term back pain. Often the person does not even realize that he or she is actually depressed. The following questionnaire will help you determine if depression is playing a role in your back-pain problem. It is based on the symptoms of depression as presented in the last chapter. Again do not be tempted to say, "Yes, but if the pain were gone, I wouldn't be depressed." That may or may not be true, as we have seen in previous examples. Often once the depression and/or anxiety is set in motion, even after the pain resolves, the emotional distress continues. Further, we must look at the levels of depression and anxiety in and of themselves, as they can impact on the perception of the back pain.

Back Pain and Depression

For each of the following symptoms circle the number that best indicates how much you have been experiencing this type of feeling over the past one to two weeks. Make sure you answer all the questions. If you feel unsure about any, put down your best guess.

(continued on next page)

Back Pain and Depression *(continued)*

0 = Not at all   2 = Moderately
1 = Somewhat   3 = A lot

1. Have you been feeling sad, low, blue, or un-happy? 0 1 2 3
2. Do you feel hopeless or discouraged about the future? 0 1 2 3
3. Do you feel useless or like a failure? 0 1 2 3
4. Do you feel inadequate or inferior to others? 0 1 2 3
5. Do you feel guilty or blame yourself for everything? 0 1 2 3
6. Are you finding it difficult to make decisions? 0 1 2 3
7. Have you been feeling frustrated and irritable? 0 1 2 3
8. Have you lost interest in other people or activities? 0 1 2 3
9. Do you feel unmotivated and find it difficult to do things? 0 1 2 3
10. Do you think you're looking old, unattractive, or ugly? 0 1 2 3
11. Have you lost your appetite or had a change in weight not due to dieting? 0 1 2 3
12. Do you have trouble falling asleep, wake up during the night, or wake up earlier than you would like? 0 1 2 3
13. Do you feel tired much of the time? 0 1 2 3
14. Have you had crying spells or felt like crying but couldn't? 0 1 2 3
15. Have you lost your interest in sex? 0 1 2 3
16. Do you worry often about your general health even beyond the back-pain problem? 0 1 2 3
17. Do you have thoughts about killing yourself or do you think you might be better off dead?* 0 1 2 3

Add up your total score for the seventeen symptoms and record it here:_____

The total score will be somewhere between 0 (answering "not at all" to each item) and 51 (answering "a lot" for each item). Use the following key to interpret your score:

Total Score	Degree of Depression
0–5	Minimal or no depression
6–11	Borderline depression
12–21	Mild depression
22–31	Moderate depression
32–51	Severe depression*

* If you have had thoughts about killing yourself or scored in the severe range of depression, you should consult a qualified mental health professional.

If you have suffered from back pain for quite some time, or if your back pain is significantly interfering with your life activities, do not be surprised at the depression score that you obtain. Depression often occurs in conjunction with back pain and makes it worse. More about this topic will be discussed in a later section.

ANXIETY

As discussed previously, anxiety can range from nervousness to full panic attacks. Anxiety often begins in the subacute stage of back pain and can make pain significantly worse due to increased muscle tension. The following self-assessment questionnaire will help you determine your level of anxiety:

Back Pain and Anxiety

Instructions. The following is a list of symptoms that people sometimes have in conjunction with back pain. For each of the symptoms circle the number that best indicates how much this type of feeling has been bothering you during the past week.

(continued on next page)

Back Pain and Anxiety *(continued)*

0 = Not at all   **2 = Moderately**
1 = Somewhat   **3 = A lot**

ANXIOUS THOUGHTS AND FEELINGS

1. Anxiety, nervousness, worry, fear, or apprehension 0 1 2 3
2. Feeling that things around you are strange or unreal 0 1 2 3
3. Feeling detached from all or part of your body 0 1 2 3
4. Sudden unexpected panic episodes 0 1 2 3
5. A sense of impending doom or that something bad is about to happen 0 1 2 3
6. Feeling tense, stressed, or "uptight" 0 1 2 3
7. Difficulty concentrating 0 1 2 3
8. Racing thoughts or having your mind jump from one thing to the next 0 1 2 3
9. Frightening thoughts, fantasies, or daydreams 0 1 2 3
10. Feeling like you're about to lose control 0 1 2 3
11. Fears of going crazy 0 1 2 3
12. Fears of fainting or passing out 0 1 2 3
13. Fears of being alone or abandoned 0 1 2 3
14. Fears of criticism or disapproval 0 1 2 3

PHYSICAL SYMPTOMS

15. Skipping, racing, or pounding of the heart 0 1 2 3
16. Pain, pressure, or tightness in the chest 0 1 2 3
17. Tingling or numbness in the toes, fingers, or around the mouth 0 1 2 3
18. Butterflies, upset, or discomfort in the stomach 0 1 2 3
19. Constipation or diarrhea 0 1 2 3
20. Restlessness or jumpiness 0 1 2 3
21. Tight, tense muscles 0 1 2 3
22. Sweating not brought on by heat 0 1 2 3
23. A lump in the throat 0 1 2 3
24. Trembling or shaking 0 1 2 3
25. Rubbery or "jelly" legs 0 1 2 3
26. Feeling dizzy, light-headed, or off-balance 0 1 2 3

(continued on next page)

Back Pain and Anxiety *(continued)*

27.	Shallow breathing or "gulping" air when you breathe	0 1 2 3
28.	Cold and clammy hands	0 1 2 3
29.	Hot or cold spells	0 1 2 3
30.	Feeling tired or easily exhausted	0 1 2 3
31.	Your voice trembling when you speak	0 1 2 3

Add up your total score for the thirty-one symptoms:_____

After you have completed the anxiety questionnaire, add up your total score for all of the symptoms. Your score will range somewhere from 0 (answering "not at all" to all of the questions) to 93 (if you answered "a lot" to all symptoms). The following key will help determine your level of anxiety.

Total Score	Degree of Anxiety
0–5	Minimal or no anxiety
6–11	Borderline anxiety
12–21	Mild anxiety
22–31	Moderate anxiety
32–51	Severe anxiety
52–93	Extreme anxiety or panic

The above total score can be useful for determining how much anxiety may be contributing to your back-pain problem. Again a common response we hear is that "Well, if I didn't have the back pain, I wouldn't be anxious." That is well understood and accepted by researchers and back-pain doctors. Still the anxiety (regardless of the cause) can make your back pain worse. If the back pain is the cause of the anxiety, then the more anxiety in response to the back pain, the greater the back pain will be. This operates in a vicious, never-ending cycle unless the anxiety is addressed directly.

The result of the anxiety questionnaire can also be useful to determine how your anxiety expresses itself. In the anxiety questionnaire there are two categories of symptoms of anxiety. These include "Anxious Thoughts and Feelings" and "Physical Symptoms." You can visually scan your scores in each category to see if you express anxiety more through thoughts and feelings or through physical symptoms. This can help you realize how the anxiety is affecting you and how you can work to change it. For those of you who want even more precise information, you can determine your average score for each of the two categories. For "Anxious Thoughts and Feelings" add the total of all responses and divide the number by 14 to get the average. For "Anxious Physical Symptoms" add the total and divide by 17 to obtain the average. You can then compare the two average scores to see if your anxiety is expressed more in a particular way. Most back-pain patients will have a higher average number for "Physical Symptoms."

ANGER

Anger is commonly a part of back pain and just as commonly unrecognized. Further, it is often unrecognized by the doctor as well as by the patient. Anger can make back pain worse, prevent treatments from being effective, and increase depression and anxiety. This often goes on completely out of the awareness of the person.

Dr. Raymond Novaco has developed the Novaco Anger Inventory, shown here in abbreviated form, which will help you assess the degree of anger you may be experiencing.

Anger Inventory

Instructions. Read the following twenty-five potentially up-setting situations described below. After each situation estimate the degree to which it would provoke or anger you, using the following scale:

0 = You would feel little or no annoyance
1 = You would feel a little irritated
2 = You would feel moderately upset
3 = You would feel quite angry
4 = You would feel very angry

As you describe how you would react to each of the following situations, make your best guess about the level of irritation/anger you would experience even though details are omitted.

1. You unpack an appliance you have just bought, plug it in, and discover it doesn't work. 0 1 2 3 4
2. You're overcharged by a repairman who has you over a barrel. 0 1 2 3 4
3. You are singled out for correction, when the actions of others go unnoticed. 0 1 2 3 4
4. You get your car stuck in the mud or snow. 0 1 2 3 4
5. You are talking to someone and he or she doesn't answer you. 0 1 2 3 4
6. Someone pretends to be something he is not. 0 1 2 3 4
7. While you are struggling to carry four cups of coffee to your table at a cafeteria, someone bumps into you, spilling the coffee. 0 1 2 3 4
8. You have hung up your clothes, but someone knocks them to the floor and fails to pick them up. 0 1 2 3 4
9. You are hounded by a salesperson from the moment you walk into a store. 0 1 2 3 4
10. You have made arrangements to go somewhere with a person who backs off at the last minute and leaves you hanging. 0 1 2 3 4

(continued on next page)

Anger Inventory *(continued)*

11. You are joked about or teased.   0 1 2 3 4

12. Your car is stalled at a traffic light and the guy behind you keeps blowing his horn.   0 1 2 3 4

13. You accidentally make a wrong turn in a parking lot. As you get out of your car, someone yells at you, "Where did you learn to drive?"   0 1 2 3 4

14. Someone makes a mistake and blames it on you.   0 1 2 3 4

15. You are trying to concentrate, but a person near you is tapping his or her foot.   0 1 2 3 4

16. You lend someone an important book or tool, and he or she fails to return it.   0 1 2 3 4

17. You have had a busy day, and the person you live with starts to complain about how you forgot to do something you agreed to do.   0 1 2 3 4

18. You are trying to discuss something important with your mate or partner, who isn't giving you a chance to express your feelings.   0 1 2 3 4

19. You are in a discussion with someone who persists in arguing about a topic he or she knows very little about.   0 1 2 3 4

20. Someone sticks his or her nose into an argument between you and someone else.   0 1 2 3 4

21. You need to get somewhere quickly, but the car in front of you is going 25 mph in a 40 mph zone, and you can't pass.   0 1 2 3 4

22. You step on a gob of chewing gum.   0 1 2 3 4

23. You are mocked by a small group of people as you pass them.   0 1 2 3 4

24. In a hurry to get somewhere, you tear a good pair of slacks on a sharp object.   0 1 2 3 4

25. You use your last quarter to make a phone call but are disconnected before you finish dialing and the quarter is lost.   0 1 2 3 4

Add up your total score for the twenty-five situations:_____

Your total score will fall somewhere between 0 (answering "no annoyance" to all of the items) to 100 (answering "very angry" to all of the items). Use the following key to determine what your total anger score means.

Total Score	Degree of Anger
0–45	*Very Low Anger.* You have a very low level of anger and annoyance. Are you sure you are that relaxed?
46–55	*Low Anger.* You are more peaceful than the average person.
56–75	*Average Anger.* You experience an average amount of anger.
76–85	*Substantial Anger.* You frequently react with anger at a level far above the average person.
86–100	*Intense Anger.* You are plagued by frequent intense, furious reactions that do not quickly disappear. Your anger may often get out of control.

Anger, both direct and indirect, can have a profound impact on a person's back pain. The preceding assessment will help you determine the degree to which anger might be affecting your pain and disability.

Source: The Abbreviated Novaco Anger Inventory © 1975. Used by permission of Raymond Novaco, Ph.D., from *Anger Control:* The Development and Evaluation of An Experimental Treatment, Lexington, MA: D.C. Heath.

DISABILITY

As you may well know, back pain can have a significant impact on a person's life, resulting in some level of disability. As we have seen throughout this book, and has been documented in research, very often the level of disability does not correlate with the physical findings. We see many patients who have very few findings (e.g., a slight disc bulge, sprain-strain, or no findings at all) and are so disabled they cannot work. Alternatively we also see patients with horrendous physical findings who have minimal symptoms and are showing very little disability. Hopefully this book has given you an understanding of why this occurs. It relates to the "nonphysical" aspects of pain we have been discussing and assessing in this chapter and the previous one. Armed with that understanding, you can begin to take action to get your back pain and your life under control.

It is useful to determine just how much your back pain is affecting your life. In this way you and your doctor can begin to focus on areas that need to change and you will be able to assess your progress. Assessing your level of disability throughout your treatment will also help you determine whether you are benefiting from the treatment or not. As we have discussed, many treatment approaches actually result in more disability and suffering.

One of the best measures of this type is the Roland and Morris Disability Questionnaire. Please complete the following:

Disability

When your back hurts, you may find it difficult to do some of the things you normally do.

Following are some sentences that people have used to describe themselves when they have back pain. When you read them, you may find that some stand out because they describe you *today*. As you read the list, think of yourself *today*. When you read a sentence that describes you today, circle "Yes." If that sentence does not describe you today, circle "No." Remember, only answer yes if you are sure the sentence describes you today.

1. I stay home most of the time because of my back.   Yes No
2. I change position frequently to try to get my back comfortable.   Yes No
3. I walk more slowly than usual because of my back.   Yes No
4. Because of my back I am not doing any of the jobs that I usually do around the house.   Yes No
5. Because of my back I use the handrail to get upstairs.   Yes No

---

(continued on next page)

Disability *(continued)*

6. Because of my back I lie down to rest more often.   **Yes No**
7. Because of my back I have to hold on to something to get out of an easy chair.   **Yes No**
8. Because of my back I try to get other people to do things for me.   **Yes No**
9. I get dressed more slowly than usual because of my back.   **Yes No**
10. I only stand up for short periods of time because of my back.   **Yes No**
11. Because of my back I try not to bend or kneel down.   **Yes No**
12. I find it difficult to get out of a chair because of my back.   **Yes No**
13. My back is painful almost all of the time.   **Yes No**
14. I find it difficult to turn over in bed because of my back.   **Yes No**
15. My appetite is not very good because of my back pain.   **Yes No**
16. I have trouble putting on my socks (or stockings) because of the pain in my back.   **Yes No**
17. I only walk short distances because of my back pain.   **Yes No**
18. I sleep less well because of my back pain.   **Yes No**
19. Because of my back pain I get dressed with help from someone else.   **Yes No**
20. I sit down for most of the day because of my back.   **Yes No**
21. I avoid heavy jobs around the house because of my back.   **Yes No**
22. Because of my back pain I am more irritable and bad-tempered with people than usual.   **Yes No**
23. Because of my back I go upstairs more slowly than usual.   **Yes No**
24. I stay in bed most of the time because of my back.   **Yes No**

Add up all items answered "Yes" and record the total here:_____

Source: Roland and Morris Disability Questionnaire © 1983 by Harper & Row. Used by permission of J. B. Lippincott, Philadelphia, PA.

On this questionnaire the higher your score, the more your back pain is causing disability. It can be useful to take the disability questionnaire periodically as you apply the principles outlined in this book and get the proper treatment for your back pain. If the process is working, you should see less and less disability as you get better.

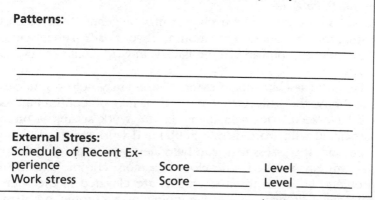

THE BACK-PAIN ASSESSMENT GRID

Using the questionnaires previously presented, you can get a good idea of all aspects of your back-pain problem. You can summarize your findings on the Back-Pain Assessment Grid. This grid has five sections: Patterns, External Stress, Internal Stress, Physical Stress (Disability), and Self-destructive Behaviors.

In the Patterns section of the assessment fill in any patterns to your pain, activities, or emotions that you discovered from the PAMM diary. In the External Stress section fill in your scores from the SRE (page 290) and the work-stress assessment (page 295). After each score fill in the level that corresponds to the score (e.g.: low, moderate, high). Do the same for the Internal Stress measures of depression, anxiety, and anger (pages 297–303). In the Physical Stress section fill in your score from the Roland and Morris Disability Questionnaire (page 306). In the Self-destructive Behaviors section answer the questions as honestly as you can in terms of increase in behaviors that you know are not healthy for you.

Patterns:

_____

_____

_____

_____

External Stress:
Schedule of Recent Experience   Score _____   Level _____
Work stress   Score _____   Level _____

(continued on next page)

THE BACK-PAIN ASSESSMENT GRID *(continued)*

Internal Stress:

Depression	Score _____	Level _____
Anxiety	Score _____	Level _____
Anger	Score _____	Level _____

Physical Stress:

Roland and Morris Disability Questionnaire	Score _____	

Self-destructive Behaviors

Increase in alcohol use	Yes	No
Starting (or increase) smoking	Yes	No
Medication overuse	Yes	No
Weight gain or loss	Yes	No
Other_____	Yes	No

Interpretation of the Back-Pain Assessment Grid

The interpretation of the Back-Pain Assessment Grid is very straightforward. Simply scan the findings to help you understand the many aspects of your back-pain problem that may need to be addressed. Depending on the phase of back pain you are experiencing, interpretation and use of the grid may be different.

Acute Back Pain

As you may recall, acute back pain may be generally defined as lasting less than about three months. If your back pain falls into this category, you can use the Back-Pain Grid results in several ways.

First, the assessments of external stress may help you understand how the pain started and why it may be continuing. As we have seen, back-pain injury in the work setting is often associated with work dissatisfaction and work stress.

Second, the assessment can help alert you to the possibility that you are at risk for developing a more chronic back-pain problem. If any of the assessments are elevated in the acute pain stage, it may be the beginning of a chronic problem.

These areas should be addressed quickly and aggressively, as outlined in this book. This will help you avoid becoming a "back-pain patient."

Recurrent Acute Back Pain

Recurrent acute back pain is back pain that "comes and goes," often staying for weeks or months at a time and then "goes away" for a time. The assessment grid can help you determine what triggers might be causing the pain to begin. These might be an emotional state, stress, deconditioning, or some other influences. Once you understand this, you can take action to prevent the back pain from happening in the future. In addition the assessment grid can help you see how you deal with these occurrences and what will help you get over them more quickly.

Chronic Back Pain

As with the other categories of back pain, the assessment grid can help you (and your doctor or other health care provider) understand and monitor all aspects of the problem. In chronic back pain, if all elements of the problem are not addressed, then improvement is less likely.

Presurgical Screening or Preparation for Spine Surgery

If you and your doctor have decided that you are an appropriate surgical candidate (hopefully using the guidelines in this book), the assessment grid can help in many ways. First it can help determine if you are ready for surgery or if certain things need to be checked prior to surgery. If external and internal stressors are high, there is overuse of alcohol and pain medications, and physical deconditioning exists, a preparation for surgery is probably appropriate. This might include decreasing medications, increasing physical conditioning, and addressing the stressors.

Stress-Related Back Pain

The grid can also help you understand how emotions may be impacting on your level of pain and disability. If these indicators are elevated and there are a lack of physical findings to explain the pain, it will be important to investigate emotional issues. This will help you avoid unnecessary and possibly harmful treatment as well as putting you on the proper road to recovery.

CHAPTER 16

TAKING RESPONSIBILITY FOR OVERCOMING YOUR BACK PAIN

Why is it that one person with back pain will successfully over-come it and another person, with the very same condition, will suffer endlessly? We believe it is because of two reasons. One is getting the right kind of treatment, as discussed throughout this book. The other is how well the person takes responsibil-ity for improving his or her quality of life while coping with the pain. This latter issue is subsumed under five areas:

- **Your attitudes and thoughts**
- **Your willingness to put in the effort to get better**
- **Your purpose and sense of meaning in life**
- **Your ability to establish goals for yourself and plans to attain them**
- **Your courage and willingness to overcome fears**

In the following pages we will rely on the wisdom of others to underscore how important it is that you pay attention to these areas. You can use the following truths to help you overcome back-pain suffering so that you may live your life as you choose.

Your Attitudes and Thoughts

People can alter their lives by altering their attitudes.
—*William James*

Whether you think you can or think you can't—you are right.
                                    —*Henry Ford*

If you've made up your mind you can do something, you're absolutely right.   —*Unknown*

Many receive advice, only the wise profit from it.
                                        —*Syrus*

Life will always be to a large extent what we ourselves make.   —*Samuel Smiles*

These tenets support our discussion of how your thoughts influence your emotions, your perception of back pain, and virtually all aspects of your life.

Your Willingness to Put in the Effort to Get Better

About the only thing that comes without effort is old age.   —*Unknown*

It's the constant and determined effort that breaks down all resistance, sweeps away all obstacles.
                                —*Claude M. Bristol*

Plan your work for today and every day, then work your plan.   —*Norman Vincent Peale*

In the middle of difficulty lies opportunity.
                                —*Albert Einstein*

Our greatest glory is not in never falling, but in rising every time we fall.   —*Confucius*

Never, never, never quit.   —*Winston Churchill*

Getting over your back pain through physical and mental reconditioning takes individual, personal effort. In most medical treatments the doctor does something to you and you are a passive recipient. The way to overcome most back pain is just the opposite. Get involved in a physical reconditioning program, pay attention to emotional factors, and keep up the effort.

Your Purpose and Sense of Meaning in Life

Purpose is what gives life meaning. —*Unknown*

The indispensable first step to getting the things you want out of life is this: decide what you want.
—*Ben Stein*

A man without a purpose is like a ship without a rudder. —*Thomas Carlyle*

When you cease to make a contribution, you begin to die. —*Eleanor Roosevelt*

Whether you have been suffering from back pain for weeks, months, or years, it is important to have purpose and meaning in your life beyond the pain. We find the patients who do best are those who do not allow the pain to become the center of their lives. The more purpose and meaning you have in other areas of your life, the less the back pain will impact upon you negatively.

Your Ability to Establish Goals for Yourself and Plans to Attain Them

The most important thing about goals is having one.
—*Geoffrey F. Abert*

People with goals succeed because they know where they're going. —*Earl Nightingale*

If you only care enough for a result, you will most certainly attain it. —*William James*

A good goal is like a strenuous exercise—it makes you stretch. —*Mary Kay Ash*

> Obstacles are those frightful things you see when you take your eyes off your goals.
> —*Unknown*

An essential element in successfully overcoming your back pain is having concrete goals. In our work we help patients establish goals related to their back pain as well as to any and all other areas of their lives. Goals can be developed in any area of your life, including such diverse areas as your exercise program, employment, recreational activities, financial status, relationships, and sex life.

Your Courage and Willingness to Overcome Fears

> All glory comes from daring to begin.
> —*Eugene F. Ware*

> Courage is resistance to fear, mastery of fear—not absence of fear.
> —*Mark Twain*

> Don't be afraid to take a big step if one is indicated. You can't jump across a chasm in two small jumps.
> —*David Lloyd George*

> Courage is doing what you're afraid to do. There can be no courage unless you're scared.
> —*Eddie Rickenbacher*

> Act as though it were impossible to fail. —*Unknown*

> Failure is not the worst thing in the world. The very worst is not to try.
> —*Unknown*

Developing a plan for recovery, facing your fears of the pain, and following through on your plan takes courage and a commitment to try. This decision and follow-through can only be done by you, with health care professionals providing the guidance. This commitment will allow you to overcome suffering from back pain.

GLOSSARY

Acetaminophen. The active pain-relieving ingredient in Tylenol.

Acupuncture. A treatment technique based on ancient Chinese medicine principles in which small needles are placed at specific body locations to cause a therapeutic benefit (e.g., pain relief).

Acute back pain. Back pain that is severe and/or of relatively short duration; to be contrasted with *chronic back pain.*

Addiction. A psychological craving for a drug or substance. It includes aspects of tolerance and dependence. Research now shows that a very small percentage of pain patients who take pain medicines will become addicted, although they will develop dependence and tolerance.

Aerobic exercise. Any exercise that stimulates and strengthens the heart and lungs, improving the body's use of oxygen.

Affect. In medicine this refers to the emotions.

Analgesic. Any medication that is primarily used for pain relief.

Anesthetic. A drug that is used to abolish the sensation of pain.

Ankylosing spondylitis. An inflammatory disease of the spine that is progressive. It is more common in men.

Annulus. The fibrous outer portion of the spinal discs, which are between the vertebrae.

Anterior. Situated in front of or in the forward part of an organ.

Antianxiety Medication. Also termed anxiolytics; medications that are used primarily for the relief of anxiety.

Antidepressants. Medications that are developed to treat depression. They are also used in pain conditions, but at lower dosage ranges.

Anti-inflammatory. Medication that decreases inflammation, swelling, and pain. Examples include Motrin, Naprosyn, and aspirin.

Arachnoiditis. An inflammation of the connective tissues (the spinal arachnoid) around the spinal cord. *Arachnoid* literally means "like a cobweb," and this is how the structure looks on imaging studies.

Arthritis. Inflammation of a joint that can be accompanied by swelling and pain.

Arthrodesis. A surgical procedure that is more commonly termed a fusion.

Babinski's test. A test for central nervous system (brain and spinal cord) disease. The sole of the foot is scratched and the reflexive response of the toes can help determine if disease is present.

Benign. Literally means "kindly"; not malignant or dangerous, and favorable for recovery.

Bilateral. Having two sides, or pertaining to both sides.

Biofeedback. A process whereby a physical system (e.g., muscle tension, blood pressure, heart rate, sweat-gland activity) is measured by sophisticated equipment for the purposes of bringing it under the person's voluntary control.

Black-and-white thinking. A type of irrational thinking in which everything is analyzed in terms of polar opposites.

Blaming. A negative type of thinking in which the person with back pain makes something or someone else responsible. This can significantly impede getting better.

Bone scan. A special X ray of the body that is done after a radioactive dye is injected and allowed to concentrate in the skeleton. Areas of increased concentration of activity (due to increased blood flow) are significant. The primary use is to diagnose infection, tumor, fracture, or arthritis of the bones.

Bone spurs. See *Osteophytes.*

Bulging disc. A disc (which is between the vertebrae) that protrudes from its normal space and may or may not cause any symptoms.

Bursitis. An inflammation of the bursa, which is the lubricating structure within a joint.

Catastrophizing. A type of irrational thinking in which the worst possible future scenario is developed and then acted upon as if it will actually happen.

Cervical spine. The portion of the spine that comprises the neck. It is made up of seven vertebrae.

Chemonucleosis. A process in which a substance is injected into the disc to dissolve a portion of it that may be causing symptoms. This process is no longer used in the United States due to problems. (See also *Chymopapain.*)

Chiropractor. A practitioner trained in spinal manipulation. Chiropractors receive a D.C. degree (doctor of chiropractic).

Chronic back pain. This has typically been defined as back pain that goes beyond three to six months' duration. It might also be defined as "pain beyond the point of tissue healing." It is commonly also termed chronic benign back pain.

Chymopapain. Extracted from the papaya fruit, this substance is often used to dissolve the ruptured portion of a disc in the chemonucleolysis procedure.

Claudication. Limping; symptoms characterized by the absence of pain in a limb at rest with increased pain and weakness after walking has begun.

Coccydynia. Literally pain in the coccyx or tailbone area.

Coccyx. The "tailbone"; the small bone at the end of the sacrum.

Cognitive/cognition. A thought or related to the process of thinking.

Cryotherapy. Literally means "treatment utilizing cold."

CT scan or CAT scan. Literally stands for "computerized (axial) tomography." A computerized X-ray recording of "slices," or sections, of the body.

Deconditioning syndrome. Also termed the disuse syndrome. It can be separated into mental and physical deconditioning. It refers to the negative result of "resting" the body (due to back pain) over time.

Degeneration. Deterioration; a progressive change of cells or tissue to a level of less function and increased impairment. Commonly used to describe changes in the disc.

Degenerative disc disease. Any disease that causes changes in the disc space with loss of tissue and height. This may be a finding on imaging studies and occur with or without symptoms.

Dependence (drug). This refers to the fact that if pain medicines have been used for an extended period of time and are suddenly stopped, withdrawal symptoms will occur. (See *Addiction* and *Tolerance*.)

Diathermy. A technique for generating heat below the surface of the skin, typically through the use of electric current.

Disc (intervertebral). Cartilage tissue that separates the spinal vertebrae and acts as a shock absorber. Each disc has two main parts: the outer ring (annulus fibrosus) and the inner ring (nucleus pulposus). The disc is made up of 80 percent water.

Disc degeneration. The process whereby the discs lose water and shrink in size. This occurs most commonly as part of the normal aging process and may or may not cause symptoms. Often used interchangeably with *degenerative disc disease,* which is often an inaccurate term.

Discectomy. The surgical removal of all or part of a disc (usually in the case of a herniated disc).

Disc narrowing. When a disc has degenerated to the point of narrowing the distance between the vertebrae above and below.

Discography. Also termed *discogram;* a test that includes injecting a radioactive dye into the disc. It is done for two purposes: to get a CT image of the spine with the dye and to determine whether the injection of the dye reproduces the patient's pain.

Dorsal. Pertaining to a position more toward the back surface; the same as *posterior.*

Dura. Also termed the *dura mater;* the tough, protective, outermost membrane covering the spinal cord and brain.

Electrodiagnostic studies. Any test in which electricity is used to test nerve function. The most common of these are nerve conduction studies and electromyography (EMG).

Endorphins. Natural painkillers, which are released by the brain.

Entitlement. The belief or attitude that "somebody or something owes me something for the pain I am experiencing." This is associated with the belief that humans are owed a pain-free existence. It can be a great obstacle to improvement.

Epidural injection. The introduction of anesthetic into the epidural space.

Epidural space. The space just outside the dura. It lies between the dura and the vertebrae.

Ergonomics. The study of the use of the body in various situations, including work, sports, and other settings. It is the interaction between the body and the environment.

Exercise physiologist. A practitioner who has been trained in proper exercise approaches.

Extension. Bending the spine backward.

Facet joints. The joints located behind the vertebral body that connect the posterior ("toward the back") aspects of the vertebrae.

Failed-back-surgery syndrome. A type of chronic back pain that develops after one or more spine surgeries that are not successful in relieving the symptoms.

Fibromyalgia. A diagnosis that includes characteristic points of muscle tenderness along with sleep disturbance, fatigue, and diffuse pain.

Filtering. A type of irrational thinking in which all positive aspects of a situation are excluded ("filtered") so that only the negative elements are left.

Flexion. Bending the spine in a forward direction.

Foramina. An opening through a bone or membrane for the passage of a nerve.

Functional-restoration program. A multidisciplinary approach that emphasizes progressively increasing function. (See also *work-hardening program* and *pain clinic*.)

Functional-restoration treatment. A multidisciplinary treatment program for back pain that focuses on progressive physical and mental reconditioning.

Fusion. The act or process of "melting" together; a spinal fusion is a surgical procedure whereby bone grafts are placed in between two or more vertebrae and allowed to grow together. This reduces mobility in that part of the spine.

Fusion with instrumentation. A fusion in which metal rods or plates are used to help secure the vertebrae together.

Gate-control theory of pain. The theory that postulates that there are "nerve gates" in the spinal cord that can open (more pain) and close (less pain) due to a variety of factors.

Hemilaminectomy. The surgical removal of a vertebral lamina on only one side.

Herniated disc. Protrusion of the nucleus of a disc through the annulus fibrosus (outer ring). This condition produces symptoms (e.g., pain down the leg) when the disc material irritates or compresses a nerve.

Hydrotherapy. Literally means any therapy or treatment that utilizes water.

Hypochondriasis. A preoccupation with the body and irrational fear of presumed illness.

Iatrogenic. A condition that is brought on or worsened by a doctor's recommendation or treatment. Many problems with back pain are often iatrogenic.

Idiopathic back pain. Back pain without a well-known or identifiable cause. Research indicates that most back pain is idiopathic, even though practitioners will attempt a diagnosis.

Imaging studies. A term used to denote tests such as CT scan and MRI.

Impotence. Loss of ability of the male to maintain an erection to the point of ejaculation.

Invasive treatment. Any treatment that involves penetrating the skin. To be contrasted with noninvasive, conservative treatment.

Kinesiologist. Trained in the mechanics and anatomy of movement.

Kinesophobia. Literally means the irrational fear *(phobia)* of movement *(Kineso-)*. It is implicated in the development of the disuse syndrome and chronic back pain.

Kyphosis. A curvature of the spine that bends a person forward.

Laminectomy. A surgery to remove a portion of the lamina (the part of the vertebrae just behind the spinal canal). It is usually done to relieve pressure on the spinal cord and nerves coming from it.

Laminotomy. Surgical creation of an opening in the lamina.

Lateral bending. Bending the spine to either side.

Ligament. A band of fibrous tissue that connects bones or cartilages, serving to support joints.

Lordosis. The natural forward curve of the lower spine (looking at the spine from the side).

Lumbago. An outdated term for lower back pain.

Lumbar spine. The area of the spine that comprises the lower back. It is made up of five vertebrae.

Lumbar stenosis. A narrowing (stenosis) of the spinal canal in the lumbar region. This can occur for a variety of reasons. There is a high degree of natural variability in canal size, which makes judgment of stenosis difficult.

Lumbosacral sprain/strain. An imprecise term for injury to the muscles, ligaments, or tendons of the back. Although often impossible to differentiate, *sprain* usually refers to ligament injury, whereas *strain* refers to muscle injury.

Magnetic resonance imaging (MRI). A popular imaging technique that uses a strong magnetic field rather than X ray and shows great detail of the anatomical structures.

Malingering. The voluntary production and presentation of false or grossly exaggerated symptoms in pursuit of some specific goal (e.g., compensation).

322

Manipulation. Primarily the movement of bones (e.g., the vertebrae) through the application of force by the practitioner (most often a chiropractor, osteopath, or physical therapist). Sounds or "cracking" noises are often heard, which is the releasing of gases from the joints. It may also be termed *an adjustment* or *joint mobilization.*

McKenzie exercises. A popular set of exercises that promote extension of the back.

Mind reading. Making assumptions about (and acting upon) what another person is thinking without actually knowing.

Modality. Any method or form of physical treatment; most commonly used to refer to the "passive modalities," in which the patient is a passive receiver of the treatment (e.g., hot pack, ultrasound, massage).

Muscle spasm. The involuntary contraction of muscles that cause pain. Whether it is a significant source of back pain is controversial.

Myelography (or **CT-myelogram**). An X ray and CT scan done after the injection of a radioactive dye ("contrast dye") into the spinal canal for better viewing of the structure. This test should only be done when surgery is being considered. With the advent of the newer water-soluble dyes the side effects (most notably severe headache) have been decreased.

Myositis. Literally means "inflammation of the muscles."

Nerve root. The portion of the nerve as it exits from the dura through the foramen ("opening" in the vertebrae) and just beyond the vertebrae. Several nerve roots come together to form larger nerves, such as the sciatic nerve.

Neurologic deficit. A loss of reflex, strength, or sensation.

Neurologist. A medical doctor who specializes in problems of the nervous system. Neurologists use nonsurgical treatment approaches.

Neurosurgeon. A medical doctor who specializes in problems of the nervous system utilizing a surgical treatment approach.

Nociception. The perception of a nerve (or nerve ending) system of painful stimulation due to trauma or injury.

Nucleus pulposus. The central or inner part of the disc.

Objective findings. Findings in medicine that are the designation of a symptom or condition perceptible to others besides the patient. (To be contrasted with *Subjective findings*.) For example, pain is a subjective complaint, whereas MRI results are objective findings.

Organic. Related to being physical or explainable by physical causes. In medical jargon pain is often characterized as *organic* or *functional,* where the latter term refers to a psychological or emotional basis. In modern practice this distinction is not useful and should not be made.

Orthopedist. A medical doctor who has been specially trained in problems of the skeletal system. Orthopedists' training emphasizes surgical approaches.

Osteoarthritis. A degenerative joint condition usually associated with aging. It may or may not produce symptoms.

Osteomalacia. An abnormal softening of the bone often due to vitamin deficiency.

Osteopath. A practitioner who has been trained in a system of manipulative treatments and other techniques. These doctors have a D.O. degree (doctor of osteopathy).

Osteophytes. Bony spurs that can occur on the vertebrae. They are occasionally implicated in irritating the spinal nerves.

Osteoporosis. A weakening of the bone as it loses some of its density.

Overgeneralizing. An irrational type of thinking that takes one aspect of a situation and applies it to all other situations.

Pain clinic. A multidisciplinary center that incorporates the expertise of a variety of health professionals to evaluate and treat patients in a highly coordinated fashion. These programs usually stress that the patient must take personal responsibility for getting well. (See also *Functional-restoration treatment* and *Work-hardening program.*)

Pedicle. The bony structure that connects the vertebrae to the posterior structures. It is the site of insertion for "pedicle screws," used in some fusion surgeries.

Physiatrist. A medical doctor who has specialized training in problems of the musculoskeletal system (muscles and bones). This doctor does not perform surgery and emphasizes a rehabilitation approach. This doctor is often recommended as the most appropriate to treat the majority of back-pain problems.

Physical therapist. A practitioner trained in rehabilitation. Physical therapists will generally have an RPT certification (registered physical therapist) and work under a physician's prescription.

Pinched nerve. A nonmedical term for compression of a nerve.

Placebo. A procedure or substance with no known therapeutic value but one that can still produce a positive response simply based upon the patient's belief that it will work.

Podiatrist. A practitioner who specializes in problems of the feet.

Posterior. Situated in the back of, or in the back part of, or affecting the back part of a structure. (See also *Dorsal.*)

Pseudoarthrosis. Most commonly refers to a situation in which a fusion was attempted but the healing of the bone grafts (in between the vertebrae) resulted in incomplete union.

Psychiatrist. A medical doctor who does a residency and specializes in the practice of psychiatry. Psychiatrists will often focus on medication management and should have special training for back-pain problems.

Psychological. Dealing with mental processes, emotions, and human behavior.

Psychologist. A practitioner trained in the evaluation and treatment of problems related to mental processes, emotions, and behavior. They typically hold one of three different types of doctoral degrees (Ph.D., Psy.D., Ed.D.). Specialization in pain management is increasing.

Psychosocial. Pertaining to the psychological aspects of an individual relative to his or her social surroundings.

Psychosomatic. Also *psycho-physiological;* a physical condition that results from psychological causes. This is not an "imaginary" problem. Rather there are actual physical changes due to nonphysical factors. (See *Stress-related back pain.*)

Radiculitis. Inflammation of a spinal nerve. This causes pain along the path of the nerve into the affected extremity (the arms or legs). (See *Sciatica.*)

Range of motion. The physiological range of a joint along several different axes.

Recurrent acute back pain. Episodes of back pain that are of varying duration and separated by relatively pain-free periods. It may represent the most common type of back-pain condition.

Rheumatologist. A medical doctor who specializes in arthritic problems.

Ruptured disc. (See *Herniated disc.*)

Sacroiliac (SI) joint. The joint between the sacrum and the pelvis. There are two SI joints, one on each side.

Sciatica. A common term for pain in the area of the body supplied by the sciatic nerve. This condition usually includes pain in the buttock(s) and the back of the leg(s). It is due to irritation of the sciatic nerve or nerve roots.

Scoliosis. An abnormal curve of the spine to the side. It is often very mild and usually does not cause symptoms. In severe cases it is treated with bracing or surgery. It is often inappropriately used as an excuse for manipulation treatment to "straighten" the spine.

Sedative. Any medication that is primarily used to induce sleep. Also referred to as *hypnotics.*

Specificity theory of pain. Originally proposed by Descartes, it postulates that there is a one-to-one relationship between pain and the amount of tissue damage. It has been shown to be inaccurate. (See *Gate-control theory.*)

Spinal stenosis. A "narrowing" of the spinal canal to an abnormal degree. Stenosis is classified as follows: congenital (from birth), developmental (genetic origin), and acquired (developed after birth). Acquired stenosis due to degenerative changes in the disc is most common.

Spinous processes. The bony knobs on the vertebrae to which muscles and ligaments attach.

Spondylalgia. Pain in the vertebrae.

Spondylitis. Literally means "inflammation of the vertebrae"; usually this is due to normal wear-and-tear changes associated with aging and is rarely a cause of back pain.

Spondylolisthesis. Literally means "slipping vertebrae"; it is the slipping forward of an individual vertebra relative to the one below it.

Spondylosis. Degenerative changes in the discs and the facet joints.

Sprain. An injury to the fibers of a supporting ligament of a joint.

Straight-leg raise. A test used as part of the physical examination to determine if there is irritation of the sciatic nerve.

Strain. To overexercise; the overstretching or overexertion of a muscle or muscles.

Stress-related back pain. (See also *Tension myalgia syndrome.*) Back pain that is thought to be primarily caused and maintained by psychological and emotional factors.

Subacute back pain. Back pain of six to twelve weeks' duration. It is the stage between the acute and chronic conditions.

Subjective findings. Findings in medicine that are the designation of a symptom or condition perceptible only to the patient. Pain is a subjective symptom (contrast with *Objective findings*).

Subluxation. A term commonly used by chiropractors that means "misalignment." Whether it is actually a source of back pain is highly controversial. When used by physicians, a subluxation is a partial dislocation.

Suffering. A perceived threat to one's well-being (such as the belief that debilitating back pain is imminent). It often involves anticipation of a possible threat that may or may not exist.

TENS (transcutaneous electrical nerve stimulation). A procedure whereby low levels of electricity are applied to areas of pain by electrodes placed on the skin.

Tension myalgia syndrome (TMS). Widespread muscle pain that is thought to arise due to psychological issues. Originally formulated by the Mayo Clinic.

Thoracic spine. The middle part of the back, comprising twelve vertebrae. It is the most stable part of the spine due to the attachment of the ribs. It is rarely a source of back pain.

Tolerance (drug). The biochemical process whereby the body can become accustomed to higher and higher doses of pain medicines, which then become less and less effective. (See also *Addiction* and *Dependence.*)

Traction. A procedure whereby pressure is applied to the spine in order to pull the vertebrae away from one another. Research suggests that traction is ineffective.

Ultrasound. A technique for generating heat below the surface of the skin through the use of sound waves.

Unilateral. One-sided or pertaining to only one side.

Vertebra. A bone of the spine. Each vertebra has three parts: the vertebral body, the transverse process, and the spinous process.

Vertebral canal. The tunnel that extends through the vertebrae in which the spinal cord lies.

Vertebral osteomyelitis. An infection in the vertebrae.

Work-hardening program. A multidisciplinary treatment approach that focuses on simulating the demands of the work environment as part of the rehabilitation. (See also *Functional-restoration program* and *Pain clinic.*)

X ray. A high-energy electromagnetic wave. A tissue or organ that is dense (such as bone) absorbs more X rays, which produce a relative transparency on the film.

BIBLIOGRAPHY

CHAPTER 1

Acute Low Back Problems in Adults: Assessment and Treatment. Clinical Practice Guideline, Quick Reference Guide Number 14. S. Bigos, O. Bowyer, G. Braen, et al. Rockville, Md.: U.S. Department of Health and Human Services, Public Health Service, Agency for Health Care Policy and Research, AHCPR Pub. No. 95-0643, December 1994.

"Epidemiology of Spinal Disorders." Chap. 2, pp. 10–23. J. W. Frymoyer. *Contemporary Conservative Care for Painful Spinal Disorders.* T. G. Mayer, V. Mooney, R. J. Gatchel, eds. Philadelphia: Lea and Febiger, 1991.

"The Epidemiology of Spinal Disorders." Chap. 8, pp. 107–42. G. B. J. Anderson. *The Adult Spine.* J. W. Frymoyer, editor-in-chief. New York: Raven Press, 1991.

"Quebec Task Force on Spinal Disorders: Scientific Approach to the Assessment and Management of Activity-Related Spinal Disorders." W. O. Spitzer, F. E. LeBlanc, M. Dupuis, et al. *Spine* 12 (7-Supplement) (1987):1–59.

CHAPTER 2

"Chiropractors." *Consumer Reports,* June 1994, pp. 383–90.

Smart Questions to Ask Your Doctor. D. Leeds. New York: HarperCollins, 1992.

Trust in Physician Scale (TPS). Dr. Lynda Anderson, School of Public Health, University of Michigan, 1420 Washington Heights, Ann Arbor, Mich. 48109. Used with permission.

CHAPTER 3

The Adult Spine. J. W. Frymoyer, editor-in-chief. New York: Raven Press, 1991.

Contemporary Conservative Care for Painful Spinal Disorders. T. G. Mayer, V. Mooney, R. J. Gatchel, eds. Philadelphia: Lea and Febiger, 1991.

"The Natural History of Lumbar Intervertebral Discs Extrusions Treated Non-operatively." J. A. Saal, J. S. Saal, and R. J. Herzog. *Spine* 15 (1990):683.

"Newest Knowledge of Low Back Pain: A Critical Look." A. L. Nachemson. *Clinical Orthopedics and Related Research,* no. 279 (1992):8–20.

CHAPTER 4

"Acute Versus Chronic Pain." Chap. 14, pp. 173–77. R. A. Sternbach. *Textbook of Pain.* P. D. Wall and R. Melzack, eds. New York: Churchill-Livingstone, 1984.

The Challenge of Pain. R. Melzack and P. D. Wall. New York: Basic Books, 1982.

Measurement of Subjective Responses. H. K. Beecher. New York: Oxford University Press, 1959.

"On the Relation of Injury to Pain." P. D. Wall. *Pain* 6 (1979):253–64.

"Pain Mechanisms: A New Theory." R. Melzack and P. D. Wall. *Science* 150 (1965):971–79.

"Relationship of Significance of Wound to Pain Experienced." H. K. Beecher. *Journal of the American Medical Association* 161 (1956):1609-13.

CHAPTER 5

"The Back." Chap. 5. J. E. Anderson. *Grant's Atlas of Anatomy.* Baltimore: Williams and Wilkins, 1978.

"The Back." Chap. 12, pp. 791-823. R. C. Snell. *Clinical Anatomy for Medical Students.* Boston: Little, Brown, and Co., 1981.

Clinical Neuroanatomy Made Ridiculously Simple. S. Goldberg. Jersey City, N.J.: M.P. Press, Inc., 1982.

CHAPTER 6

"The Disuse Syndrome." W. M. Bortz. *Western Journal of Medicine* 141 (1984):691-94.

"Differential Diagnosis in Low Back Pain." Chap. 11, pp. 122-30. G. S. Laros. *Contemporary Conservative Care for Painful Spinal Disorders.* T. G. Mayer, V. Mooney, R. J. Gatchel, eds. Philadelphia: Lea and Febiger, 1991.

"Early Development of Physical and Mental Deconditioning in Painful Spinal Disorders." Chap. 26, pp. 278-89. R. J. Gatchel. *Contemporary Conservative Care for Painful Spinal Disorders.* T. G. Mayer, V. Mooney, R. J. Gatchel, eds. Philadelphia: Lea and Febiger, 1991.

Mind Over Back Pain. J. Sarno. New York: Berkley, 1986.

"Natural History of Low Back Disorders." Chap. 70, pp. 1537-50. J. W. Frymoyer and A. Nachemson. *The Adult Spine.* J. W. Frymoyer, editor-in-chief. New York: Raven Press, 1991.

"The Natural History of Sciatica Associated with Disc Pathology." K. Bush, N. Cowan, D. Katz, P. Gighen. *Spine* 17 (1992):1205-12.

"Spinal Irritation." Chap. 2, pp. 25-39. E. Shorter. From *Paralysis to Fatigue: A History of Psychosomatic Illness in the Modern Era.* New York: Free Press, 1992.

"Tension Myalgia as a Diagnosis at the Mayo Clinic and Its Relationship to Fibromyalgia, and Myofascial Pain Syndrome." J. M. Thompson. *Mayo Clinic Proceedings* 65 (1990):1237-48.

"Toward an Integrated Understanding of Fibromyalgia Syndrome: I. Medical and Pathophysiological Aspects." M. D. Boissevain and G. A. McCain. *Pain* 45 (1991):227-38.

"Toward an Integrated Understanding of Fibromyalgia Syndrome: II. Psychological and Phenomenological Aspects." M. D. Boissevain and G. A. McCain. *Pain* 45 (1991):227-38.

CHAPTER 7

"Computerized Tomography (CT) and Enhanced CT of the Spine." Chap. 20, pp. 335-401. K. B. Heithoff and R. J. Herzog. *The Adult Spine.* J. W. Frymoyer, editor-in-chief. New York: Raven Press, 1991.

"CT-Discography." Chap. 22, pp. 443-56. K. Gill and R. P. Jackson. *The Adult Spine.* J. W. Frymoyer, editor-in-chief. New York: Raven Press, 1991.

"The Differential Utility of the MMPI as a Predictor of Outcome in Lumbar Laminectomy for Disc Herniation Versus Spinal Stenosis." L. D. Herron, J. Turner, S. Clancy, P. Weiner. *Spine* 11 (1986):847-50.

"The MMPI and Psychological Factors in Chronic Low Back Pain: A Review." A. W. Love and C. L. Peck. *Pain* 28 (1987):1-12.

"Myelography." Chap. 19, pp. 311-34. C. Neuville. *The Adult Spine.* J. W. Frymoyer, editor-in-chief. New York: Raven Press, 1991.

"Other Diagnostic Studies: Electrodiagnosis." Chap. 26, pp. 541-48. R. H. Glantz and S. Haldeman. *The Adult Spine.* J. W. Frymoyer, editor-in-chief. New York: Raven Press, 1991.

BIBLIOGRAPHY

"Plain Radiographs in Evaluating the Spine." Chap. 18, pp. 289-307. M. H. Liang, J. N. Katz, J. W. Frymoyer. *The Adult Spine*. J. W. Frymoyer, editor-in-chief. New York: Raven Press, 1991.

"The Spine." Chapter 4, pp. 117-92. K. B. Heithoff and J. L. Amster. *MRI of the Musculoskeletal System: A Teaching File*. J. H. Mink and A. L. Deutsch, eds. New York: Raven Press, 1990.

CHAPTER 8

"Conservative Therapy for Low Back Pain: Distinguishing Useful from Useless Therapy." R. A. Deyo. *Journal of the American Medical Association* 250 (1983):1057-62.

"The Effectiveness of Manual Therapy, Physiotherapy, and Treatment by the General Practitioner for Nonspecific Back and Neck Complaints: A Randomized Clinical Trial." B. W. Koes, L. M. Bouter, H. VanMameren, et al. *Spine* 17 (1992):28-35.

"Injection Studies: Role in Pain Definition." Chap. 25, pp. 527-40. V. Mooney. *The Adult Spine*. J. W. Frymoyer, editor-in-chief. New York: Raven Press, 1991.

"Newest Knowledge of Low Back Pain: A Critical Look." A. L. Nachemson. *Clinical Orthopedics and Related Research*, no. 279 (1992):8-20.

"Non-operative Treatment of Low Back Disorders, Differentiating Useful from Useless Therapy." Chap. 72, pp. 1567-80. R. A. Deyo. *The Adult Spine*. J. W. Frymoyer, editor-in-chief. New York: Raven Press, 1991.

"Spinal Manipulative Therapy in the Management of Low Back Pain." Chap. 73, pp. 1581-95. S. Haldeman and R. B. Phillips. *The Adult Spine*. J. W. Frymoyer, editor-in-chief. New York: Raven Press, 1991.

CHAPTER 9

"Efficacy of Multidisciplinary Pain Treatment Centers: A Meta-analytic Review." H. Flor, T. Fydrich, D. C. Turk. *Pain* 49 (1992):221-30.

"Exercise and the Increase in Activity Level." Chap. 10, pp. 168-83. W. E. Fordyce. *Behavioral Methods for Chronic Pain and Illness.* St. Louis: Mosby, 1976.

Functional Restoration for Spinal Disorders: The Sports Medicine Approach. T. G. Mayer and R. J. Gatchel. Philadelphia: Lea and Febiger, 1988.

"Functional Restoration with Behavioral Support: A One-Year Prospective Study of Patients with Chronic Low-Back Pain." R. G. Hazard, J. W. Fenwick, S. M. Kalisch, et al. *Spine* 14 (1989):157-61.

"Non-operative Treatment of Lumbar Intervertebral Disc with Radiculopathy: An Outcome Study." J. Saal and J. Saal. *Spine* 14 (1989):431-37.

CHAPTER 10

"Alternative Therapies for the Failed Back Syndrome." Chap. 99, pp. 2069-92. H. A. Wilkinson. *The Adult Spine.* J. W. Frymoyer, editor-in-chief. New York: Raven Press, 1991.

"Chronic Opioid Therapy for Persistent Noncancer Pain: Panacea or Oxymoron?" D. C. Turk and M. C. Brody. *American Pain Society Bulletin* 1, no. 1 (1991):1-7.

"Chronic Opioid Therapy for Persistent Noncancer Pain: Can We Get Past the Bias?" R. K. Portenoy. *APS Bulletin* 1, no. 2 (1991):1-9.

"Chronic Opioid Therapy in Nonmalignant Pain." R. K. Portenoy. *Journal of Pain and Symptom Management* 55 (1990):46-62.

"Failed Back Surgery Syndrome: 5-Year Follow-up After Spinal Cord Stimulator Implantation." R. B. North, M. G. Ewend, M. T. Lawton, et al. *Neurosurgery* 28 (1991):692-99.

"Intrathecal Infusional Therapy for Intractable Pain: Patient Management Guidelines." E. S. Krames. *Journal of Pain and Symptom Management* 8 (1993):36–46.

"Spinal Cord Stimulation for Chronic, Intractable Pain: Experience Over Two Decades." R. B. North, D. H. Kidd, M. Zahcrak, et al. *Neurosurgery* 32 (1993):384–95.

"Spinal Cord Stimulation in Contemporary Pain Management: Focus and Commentaries." *American Pain Society Journal* 2 (1993):91–106.

"Treatment of Chronic Pain by Epidural Spinal Cord Stimulation: A 10-Year Experience." K. Kumar, R. Nath, G. M. Wyant. *Journal of Neurosurgery* 75 (1991):402–07.

CHAPTER 11

"About Analgesics and Alternatives." Chap. 8, pp. 132–48. R. A. Sternbach. *Mastering Pain.* New York: Ballantine Books, 1987.

"Antidepressants for the Relief of Chronic Pain: Do They Work?" K. Goodkin and C. M. Bullion. *Annals of Behavioral Medicine* 11 (1989):84–101.

"Antidepressant-Induced Analgesia in Chronic Non-malignant Pain: A Meta-analysis of 39 Placebo-Controlled Studies." P. Onghena and B. V. Van Houdenhove. *Pain* 49 (1992):205–20.

Drug Facts and Comparisons (updated monthly). Facts and Comparisons, Inc., 111 W. Port Plaza, Ste. 400, St. Louis, MO 63146-3098.

"Narcotics." Chap. 3.A.2., pp. 514–25. R. G. Teuycross. *Textbook of Pain.* P. D. Wall and R. Melzack, eds. New York: Churchill-Livingstone, 1984.

Physicians' Desk Reference. Montvale, N.J.: Medical Economics Data Production Co., 1994.

"Psychoactive Medications as Adjuncts in Functional Restoration."
Chap. 38, pp. 465–72. P. B. Polatin. *Contemporary Conservative Care for Painful Spinal Disorders.* T. G. Mayer, V. Mooney, R. J. Gatchel, eds. Philadelphia: Lea and Febiger, 1991.

"The Use of Anti-depressants in the Treatment of Chronic Pain: A Review of the Current Evidence." C. Magni. *Drugs* 42 (1991):730–48.

CHAPTER 12

"Benefits of Psychological Preparation for Surgery (Review)." M. Johnston and C. Vogele. *Annals of Behavioral Medicine* 15 (1993):245–56.

"Childhood Psychological Trauma Correlates with Unsuccessful Lumbar Spine Surgery." J. Schofferman, D. Anderson, R. Hines, G. Smith, A. White. *Spine* 17 (6-Supplemental) (1992):138–44.

"Computed Tomographic Follow-up Study of Forty-eight Cases of Nonoperatively Treated Lumbar Intervertebral Disc Herniation." J. Y. Maigne, B. Rine, B. Deligne. *Spine* 17 (1992):1071–74.

"A Concept of Illness Tested as an Improved Basis for Surgical Decisions in Low-Back Disorders." G. Waddell, E. W. Morris, M. P. Di Paola, et al. *Spine* 11 (1986):712–19.

"Cost-effectiveness Analysis of Extended Conservative Therapy Versus Surgical Intervention in the Management of Herniated Lumbar Intervertebral Disc." L. Shvartzman, E. Weingarten, H. Sherry, S. Levin, A. Persaud. *Spine* 17 (1992):176–82.

"Lumbar Disc Herniation: A Controlled, Prospective Study with Ten Years Observation." H. Weber. *Spine* 8 (1983):131–40.

"Lumbar Disc Herniation: Computed Tomography Scan Changes After Conservative Treatment of Nerve Root Compression." M. C. Delauche-Cavallier, C. Budet, J. D. Laredo, et al. *Spine* 17 (1992):927–33.

"The Natural History of Sciatica Associated with Disc Pathology." K. Bush, N. Cowan, D. Katz, P. Gighen. *Spine* 17 (1992):1205–12.

"A Prospective Study of the Importance of Psychological and Social Factors for the Outcome After Surgery in Patients with Slipped Lumbar Disc Operated Upon for the First Time." L. V. Sorensen, O. Mors, O. Skovlund. *Acta Neurochir* 88 (1987):119-25.

"Psychological Vulnerability as a Predictor for Short-Term Outcome in Lumbar Spine Surgery: A Prospective Study." P. Thorvaldsen and E. B. Sorensen. *Acta Neurochir* 102 (1990):58-61.

CHAPTER 13

"Chemonucleolysis Update." E. Nordby. *Contemporary Orthopedics* 24 (1992):82-103.

"Clinical Efficacy of Spinal Instrumentation in Lumbar Degenerative Disc Disease." J. Zucherman, K. Hsu, G. Picetti, et al. *Spine* 17 (1992):834-37.

"Morbidity and Mortality in Association with Operations on the Lumbar Spine." R. Deyo, D. Cherkin, et al. *Journal of Bone and Joint Surgery* 74 (1992):536-43.

"Multiple Spine Surgical Failures: The Value of Adjunctive Psychological Assessment." C. D. Tollison and J. R. Satterthwaite. *Orthopaedic Review* 19 (1990):1073-77.

"Patient Outcomes After Lumbar Spinal Fusions." J. A. Turner, M. Erseck, L. Herron, et al. *Journal of the American Medical Association* 268 (1992):907-11.

"Percutaneous Discectomy: A New Concept, Technique and Twelve Years Experience." S. Hijikata. *Clinical Orthopedics* 238 (1989):9-16.

"Surgery for Lumbar Spinal Stenosis: Attempted Meta-analysis of the Literature." J. A. Turner, M. Ersek, L. Herron, R. Deyo. *Spine* 17 (1992):1-8.

"Surgical Decision Making: A System Based on Classification and Symptom Chronology." Chap. 34, pp. 403-29. V. Mooney. *Contem-*

porary Conservative Care for Painful Spinal Disorders. T. G. Mayer, V. Mooney, R. J. Gatchel, eds. Philadelphia: Lea and Febiger, 1991.

"Surgical Management of Low Back Disorders." Chap. 33, pp. 383–402. S. R. Garfin and H. N. Herkowitz. *Contemporary Conservative Care for Painful Spinal Disorders.* T. G. Mayer, V. Mooney, R. J. Gatchel, eds. Philadelphia: Lea and Febiger, 1991.

CHAPTER 14

"A Definition of Pain." J. D. Loeser. *University of Washington Medicine* 7 (1980):3–4.

A New Guide to Rational Living. A. Ellis. North Hollywood, Calif.: Wilshire Books, 1975.

Behavioral Methods for Chronic Pain and Illness. W. E. Fordyce. St. Louis: Mosby, 1976.

"Characteristics of Chronic Pain Patients: Factor Analysis of the MMPI-2." W. W. Deardorff, A. F. Chino, D. W. Scott. *Pain* 54 (1993):153–58.

"Chronic Musculoskeletal Pain and Depressive Symptoms in the National Health and Nutrition Examination I. Epidemiologic Follow-up Study." G. Magni, M. Marchutti, C. Moreschi, et al. *Pain* 53 (1993):163–68.

The Chronic Pain Control Workbook. M. Catalono. New Harbinger Publications, 564 Shattuck Ave., Oakland, Calif., 1987.

"Cognitive Distortion and Psychological Distress in Chronic Low Back Pain Patients." T. W. Smith, E. W. Aberger, M. J. Follick, D. K. Ahern. *Journal of Consulting and Clinical Psychology* 54 (1986):573–75.

Cognitive Therapy and Emotional Disorders. A. T. Beck. New York: New American Library, 1979.

BIBLIOGRAPHY

Diagnostic and Statistical Manual of Mental Disorder Fourth Edition. American Psychiatric Association, 1994.

Healing Back Pain: The Mind-Body Connection. J. Sarno. New York: Warner Books, 1991.

"Pain and Suffering: A Reappraisal." W. E. Fordyce. *American Psychologist* 43 (1988):276-83.

"Psychological Factors in the Long-Term Prognosis of Chronic Low Back Pain Patients." I. Akerlind, J. O. Hornquist, P. Bjurulf. *Journal of Clinical Psychology* 48 (1992):596-606.

The Relaxation and Stress Reduction Workbook. M. Davis, M. McKay, E. R. Eshelman. Oakland, Calif.: New Harbinger, 1982.

The Road Less Traveled. M. S. Peck. New York: Simon and Schuster, 1978.

Thoughts and Feelings: The Art of Cognitive Stress Intervention. M. McKay, M. Davis, P. Fanning. Oakland, Calif.: New Harbinger, 1981.

"The Treatment of Depression in Chronic Low Back Pain: Review and Recommendations." M. J. L. Sullivan, K. Reesor, S. Mikail, R. Fisher. *Pain* 50 (1992):5-13.

CHAPTER 15

Feeling Good: The New Mood Therapy. D. D. Burns. New York: Avon Books, 1980.

"A Study of the Natural History of Back Pain, Part I: Development of a Reliable and Sensitive Measure of Disability in Low Back Pain." M. Roland and R. Morris. *Spine* 8 (1983):144.

341

We are constantly developing new materials and resources for both the health care provider and the person who suffers with back pain. If you are interested in obtaining a list of current items, or to comment on this book, please write to:

William W. Deardorff, Ph.D.
P.O. Box 9061
Calabasas, CA
91372-9061

INDEX

Index

Index